Surgery for Varicose Veins

Single Surgical Procedures **8**

A Colour Atlas of

Surgery for Varicose Veins

C. Vaughan Ruckley

W DE G

Walter de Gruyter · Berlin · New York 1984

C. Vaughan Ruckley MB, Ch. M, FRCS (Edinburgh); Consultant Surgeon, Royal Infirmary, Edinburgh and Senior Lecturer at the University of Edinburgh, Scotland

Original Publishers: Wolfe Medical Publications Ltd., · London
Exclusive co-publishers for the Federal Republic of Germany and Austria: Walter de Gruyter & Co., Genthiner Strasse 13, D-1000 Berlin 30. 1984.

Printed by Royal Smeets Offset b.v., Weert, Netherlands

Cover design: Rudolf Hübler

General Editor, Wolfe Surgical Atlases:
William F. Walker, DSc, ChM, FRCS (Eng.), FRCS (Edin.), FRS (Edin.)

CIP-Kurztitelaufnahme der Deutschen Bibliothek

Ruckley, C. Vaughan:
A colour atlas of surgery for varicose veins / C. Vaughan Ruckley. – Berlin; New York: de Gruyter, 1984.
(Single surgical procedures; 8)
ISBN 3-11-010034-7
ISBN 3-11-010035-5 (Subskr.-Pr.)
NE: GT

Contents

Introduction

Varicose vein operations are among the commonest in general surgical units. To achieve good results the surgeon must be prepared to spend ample time, not only at the operating table but also in assessing the patient beforehand. Delegation to the most junior member of the team and relegation to the end of the operating list does not offer the best prospects for the patient.

Varicosities have a natural tendency to recur and patients should be warned about this, but provided that the major sites of reflux from the deep veins into the saphenous systems have been properly interrupted, any recurrence should be trivial and readily abolished by sclerotherapy. Therefore, after operation the surgeon should be prepared to keep the patient under review for a few years so that, should there be any residual varicosities, they can be dealt with in good time. Seldom should a second operation be required for varicose veins.

Indications for surgery

The indications for operation are cosmetic, symptomatic or prophylactic. Symptoms are generally mild and, although cosmetic reasons may be to the forefront of the patient's mind, the surgeon will usually consider that he is operating to prevent or relieve the complications of chronic venous insufficiency. The term 'chronic venous insufficiency' is used to describe varicose disease with skin complications, and usually indicates incompetence *or* occlusion of deep veins in addition to the superficial and perforator incompetence.

Skin complications include pigmentation, eczema, ulceration, and contact dermatitis. Phlebitis and deep-vein thrombosis, less frequent accompaniments of varicose veins, are nevertheless real risks that may be reduced by surgery. Occasionally, severe haemorrhages occur from varicose veins. When the cosmetic indication is uppermost, especially in young women, the surgeon may have to adjust his technique to ensure that the patient is not left with conspicuous scars. This is perhaps the best indication for the stab-avulsion method (**6**) (Rivlin 1975).

In the case of varicose ulcer it is preferable to ensure that the ulcer is healed, if necessary by a period of inpatient treatment, before operating. In particularly stubborn cases, varicose-vein surgery can be combined with ulcer excision and either primary or delayed skin grafting. Although most chronic leg ulcers remain healed after properly performed varicose-vein surgery, this is not always so, especially, if as is commonly the case, there is valvular incompetence in the deep veins, and/or associated disease which impairs healing. Indeed, before operating on the veins for a patient with skin complications, it is important to consider possible aggravating or causative diseases and to treat, where appropriate. These include obesity, hypertension, arterial insufficiency, rheumatoid disease, osteoarthritis, diabetes, skin disease, vasculitis, and blood disorders. Where chronic venous insufficiency is secondary to previous deep-vein thrombosis (the post-thrombotic syndrome), permanent occlusion of deep veins should be suspected, especially if there is persistent swelling, chronic discomfort or venous claudication. In such a case, the superficial veins should not be interfered with unless patency of deep veins has been demonstrated by phlebography.

Varicosities on the foot are usually better left alone unless the cosmetic indications are strong. They are often small and numerous. In most circumstances they are hidden and supported by the patient's shoes. Some improvement can usually be expected after calf perforators have been dealt with.

If the patient has intradermal 'spider' or 'flare' varicosities there is little that can be offered. Although some improvement occasionally follows the ligation or injection of underlying perforators, the patient should not be guaranteed any benefit.

Sclerotherapy, as described by Fegan (1963), has a place but not as a direct alternative to surgery. When there is incompetence at the saphenofemoral or the saphenopopliteal junction, the benefit of sclerotherapy is at best transitory (Hobbs 1974). The ideal role for injection treatment is in the abolition of residual varicosities after surgery and in the treatment of below-knee varicosities stemming from perforator incompetence rather than saphenous reflux. In the latter instance care must be taken not to inject a large bolus of sclerosant directly into a large perforator, because its rapid passage into the deep veins may lead to deep-vein thrombosis.

When to operate

The best stage at which to operate on varicose veins is when they are sufficiently developed for the sites of incompetence (i.e. deep to superficial reflux) to be clearly evident, but before they have become extensive or skin complications supervened. In primary varicose veins this usually means early or middle adult life. It is not the author's practice to operate on the veins of elderly patients, unless there are skin complications which cannot be controlled by conservative measures. The obese patient should reduce weight before surgery is considered.

Facilities

Most varicose vein operations are performed on an inpatient basis. However, day care is appropriate for many patients provided that they do not live a long distance from the hospital (Stephens and Dudley 1961; Ruckley *et al.* 1973). This type of care is best provided in a specifically designed day-bed unit. Improvements in anaesthesia have greatly helped, including the use of spinal or local anaesthetic. Patients for day care should be screened and selected carefully, taking into account social as well as medical history. It is a particularly good system for women with young families. Such patients often neglect their veins because they are reluctant to leave the family to spend days in hospital, for what is not considered urgent surgery. Good liaison with those who are to provide the aftercare in the home, the district nurse, the family doctor and of course the relatives, is necessary. Provided that these principles are followed, a system can be developed which is popular with patients and economical for the health service (Ruckley *et al.* 1978). If day-care facilities and satisfactory liaison with community health services are not available, then a period of 48 hours or more of hospital care is usually necessary.

Preoperative assessment

Preoperative assessment must be thorough. The patient should be examined standing on a stool or platform, on a warm surface in a warm room. It is usually possible, purely on inspection, for the practised observer to judge where the main sites of incompetence are located, for each has its characteristic pattern of varicosities. Some of these are illustrated in **16** to **23.**

Percussion: tourniquet and Perthes' tests

Percussion is a useful means of plotting the venous channels, especially where the veins are well covered by subcutaneous fat.

Next tourniquet tests are used to determine whether segments of vein are filling by way of incompetent perforators, independent of reflux at a higher level. The veins are then mapped out with an indelible felt-tip marker. If it is necessary to make incisions through tissues heavily affected by chronic venous insufficiency, it is advisable to warn the patient that delayed healing is not uncommon.

Perthes' test can be useful, especially if other methods of demonstrating deep patency, such as Doppler ultrasound or phlebography, are not available. A tourniquet is placed just below the knee, after which the patient marks time vigorously or walks on a treadmill. The onset of venous claudication indicates the presence of an occluded deep-vein system. A negative test does not obviate the need for further investigation where there is doubt about deep patency. Where the facilities of a vascular laboratory are available, Doppler ultrasound and impedance or strain-gauge plethysmography can be used to assess deep-vein patency and reduce the need for phlebography. The most reliable method, however, is phlebography, and a phlebogram which demonstrated occlusion of deep veins would usually contraindicate ligations and stripping. Patients with varicose veins who need this type of investigation are exceptional. In most cases careful physical examination is all that is required.

Principles of surgery

This book is mainly devoted to a conventional dissection-ligation approach to common patterns of varicose disease. The operation of subfascial ligation for chronic venous insufficiency is included, and avulsion is dealt with briefly. The latter technique should be particularly considered if the patient is known to have a tendency to keloid scar formation, because the cosmetic results of varicose-vein surgery can occasionally be disappointing, despite careful wound closure.

An operation for varicose veins comprises a combination of all or some of the following components: a) Sapheno-femoral ligation (The Trendelenberg operation); b) Sapheno-popliteal ligation; c) Multiple ligations. The choice of each of these components depends on accurate assessment of the pattern of incompetence in the individual leg.

The frequency with which legal cases arise from damage to femoral artery or vein testifies that this is not an area for the unsupervised junior surgeon. A clear understanding of the anatomy is essential.

For surgery to the long saphenous system the patient is positioned supine and head down. The table must be capable of being tipped, so that in the event of an unexpected severe haemorrhage, the foot of the table can be elevated high and the bleeding point controlled by compression. Thus, the hazards of attempts to clamp the bleeding points with the attendant risk of damage to femoral artery or vein are avoided.

It may be necessary to turn the patient into the prone position to give access to the upper end of the short saphenous vein, or a posterior approach to subfascial ligations. If the patient is not obese and has free joint movement, then adequate access to these areas may be possible from the front with the aid of rotation of the table and pillows under the contralateral hip and shoulder.

The Trendelenberg operation

The Trendelenberg operation has as its purpose not only the interruption of reflux down the main long saphenous vein (LSV), but also the ligation of all upper thigh tributaries so that collateral channels cannot subsequently open up. Because most patients with varicose veins, whether primary or secondary, suffer from incompetence at this level, it is most important that this part of the operation should be properly done. If there is a particular feature which characterises recurrent varicose veins it is the discovery, at the second operation, that the upper end of the LSV or its tributaries have not been dealt with correctly. Probably the commonest error is to mistake a high medial or less often lateral tributary for the LSV itself. Anatomical anomalies, such as a double saphenous vein, may also give rise to difficulty for the unwary. If there is uncertainty about the anatomy, it can be a helpful guide to pass a stripper up the LSV from knee level.

Short saphenous ligation

The same attention to detail is necessary for ligation of the termination of the short saphenous vein (SSV) at the sapheno-popliteal junction. Here the surgeon must be aware of possible anatomical variations in the level at which the SSV joins the deep vein, and in the connections between the long and short systems. Indeed Hobbs (1981) has advocated the use of preoperative phlebography for this reason.

Multiple ligations

Multiple ligations may be carried out either superficial or deep to the deep fascia, the latter being reserved for ligation of perforators in the lower half of the calf in patients with severe chronic venous insufficiency, where the induration caused by chronic inflammation or lipodermatosclerosis makes accurate superficial dissection impossible. Incisions are placed with three aims in view: a) To locate and ligate perforating veins which communicate between the superficial and deep systems; b) To interrupt tributaries which drain into the long or short saphenous stems; c) To remove the most prominent of the varicosities. It is the tributaries of the saphenous veins which become varicose not the saphenous stems themselves, although the latter do develop localised saccular dilatations ('blow-outs') where incompetent channels join.

Stripping

It is also important to emphasise that perforators usually connect with the saphenous tributaries and seldom with the main stems. For this reason stripping, although it receives much prominence in the literature, is the least important part of the operation and can, without detriment, be omitted if the other components of the operation have been completed properly. In the patient who has symptoms of arterial disease or a strong family history of obliterative arterial disease, is a diabetic or a smoker, stripping should not be performed. Where, despite these reservations, the surgeon feels that stripping would be helpful, it should be performed only from a level just below the knee to the groin. This removes the part of the saphenous stem which is likely to be associated with recurrence.

Full-length strip from ankle to groin confers no proven additional benefit and adds to the morbidity of the operation, including frequent damage to the saphenar nerve. Some surgeons also like to strip the short saphenous and segments of varicose tributaries. In the author's view, this seldom adds anything of value to the outcome.

Subfascial ligation

The method of ligating perforators on the undersurface of the deep fascia (Linton 1949) should be considered when there has been chronic inflammation in the gaiter area. Attempts to dissect veins in dense, oedematous, fibrous tissue may be difficult and inimical to healing. A long incision is therefore carried straight down to and through the deep fascia. Perforators are then easily dealt with as they emerge from the muscle. If the arterial supply is interrupted over too wide an area, the procedure is apt to be followed by wound-edge necrosis. The operation is best done under tourniquet.

Postoperative care

Carefully applied graduated compression elastic bandaging is important postoperatively, especially if the patient is to be managed as an outpatient. Haematoma is the main cause of postoperative discomfort. Elastic compression ensures that this is minimised as well as encouraging obliteration of interrupted segments of veins. Knee-length elastic stockings are fitted before operation, resumed when the sutures have been removed and continued for at least three months.

Special attention should be paid to prophylaxis against venous thromboembolism, especially if there is a history of previous phlebitis, deep-vein thrombosis or pulmonary embolism. It is the author's practice to operate only on one leg at a time, so that early ambulation can be encouraged; the patients are assisted to walk to the toilet on the evening of operation and encouraged to increase their activity on subsequent days.

The exception to the policy of early mobilisation is the patient who has had extensive subfascial ligations. In this case the patient is kept resting with the leg elevated, until the wound has been inspected on the third or fourth day. If the wound is healing well the patient is mobilised, otherwise a further period of rest is required. For all patients the foot of the bed is elevated in the early postoperative period, and ankle exercises are encouraged.

Inpatients receive subcutaneous heparin, 5000 IU, twice daily until discharged. Sclerotherapy in the few patients in whom it is required, is begun around three months after operation. Regular review for two or three years or more is recommended, although it is appreciated that this is not a practical possibility in some clinics. Alternatively, the patient must be advised to report if varicosities recur, so that they can be controlled with sclerotherapy.

The long saphenous system

1

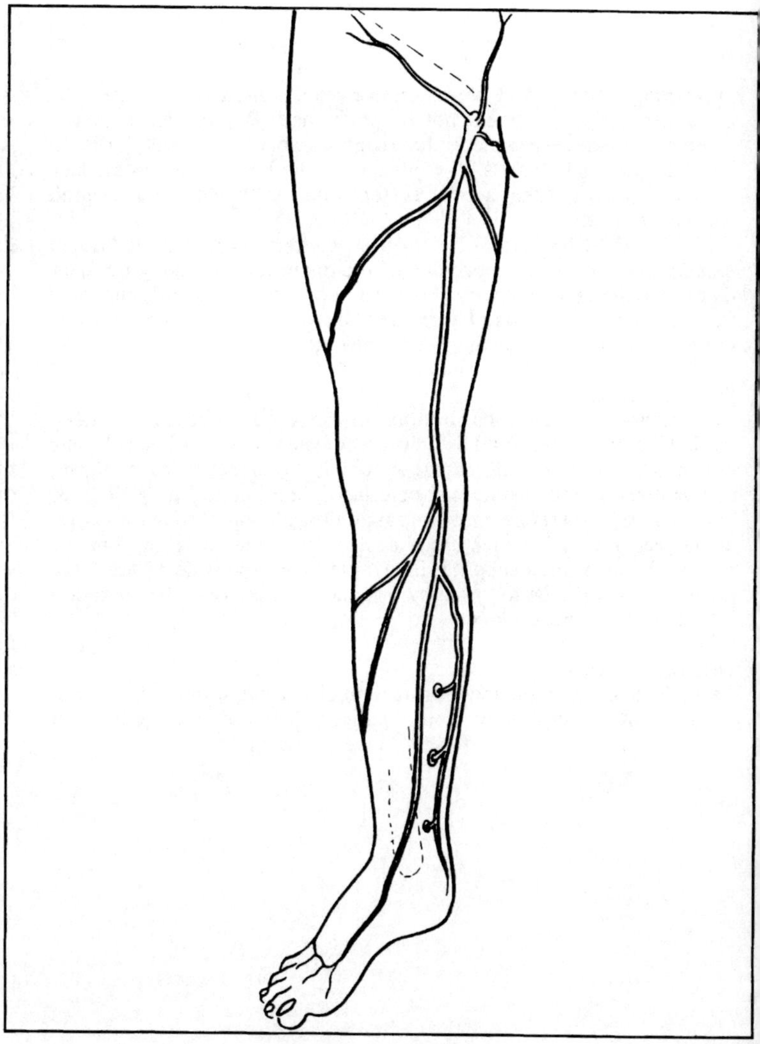

1 The long saphenous system. The long saphenous vein (LSV) begins on the dorsum of the foot from the medial end of the dorsal venous arch. It ascends crossing the tibia just above the medial malleolus from before backwards. It passes up the medial side of the calf close to the deep fascia, whereas its tributaries are more superficial. In the lower two-thirds of the calf it is accompanied by the saphenar nerve. Approximately three to four finger breadths below the line of the knee joint it is joined by the anterior-arch and posterior-arch veins. The posterior-arch vein connects with the deep veins by two or three large perforating or communicating veins at the medial border of soleus and the tendo Achilles. Perforators seldom join the saphenous veins directly. Perforators occur at other sites in the calf and thigh, but they are usually smaller and less constant in position than those of the posterior-arch vein. At knee level the LSV lies posteromedial and is more superficial. In the thigh it again lies at a deeper plane than its tributaries, as it ascends to the saphenous opening where it pierces the cribiform fascia 3 to 4 cm below and lateral to the pubic tubercle. In the upper thigh it receives an anterolateral and a posteromedial superficial femoral tributary, both of which may be large veins sometimes mistaken for the LSV itself. Just before it pierces the cribiform fascia it receives three named tributaries: the superficial external pudendal, the superficial circumflex iliac, and the superficial inferior epigastric. Entering its medial side as it passes through the fossa ovalis to join the common femoral vein is the deep external pudendal vein.

2a

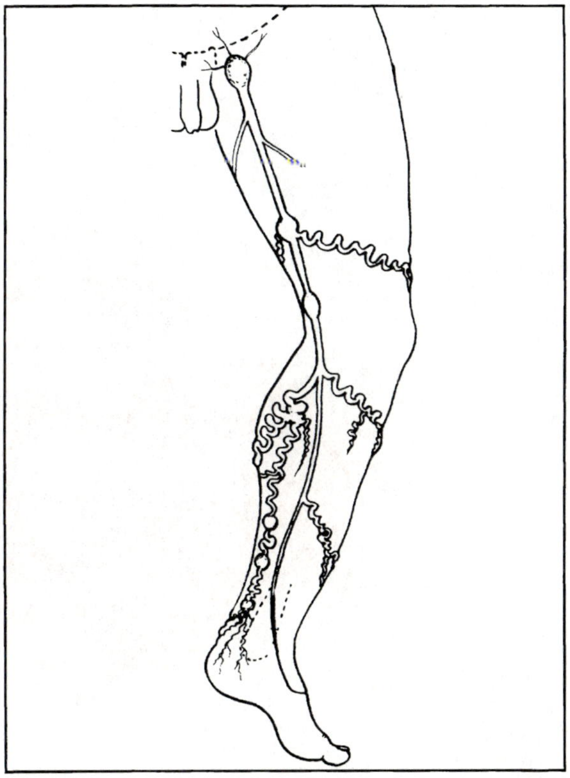

2b

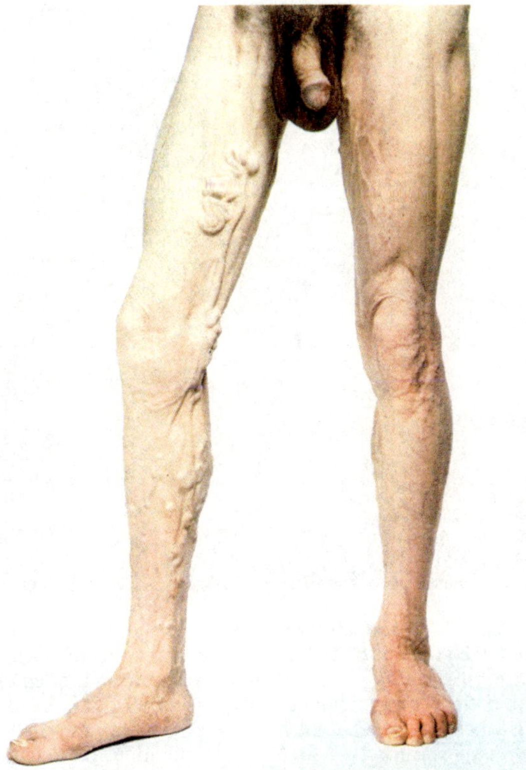

2a and b Varicosities of the long saphenous system. The tributaries of the LSV, being thinner-walled than the main stem, become dilated and tortuous i.e. varicose when subjected to back pressure. The LSV does not become tortuous but does dilate at points beyond incompetent valves and where it is joined by perforators or distended tributaries. These 'blow-outs' are readily palpable and, in the thin individual, visible.

3a

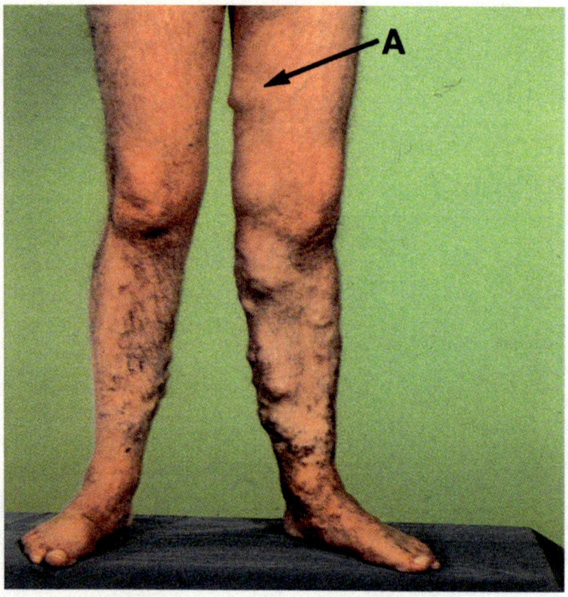

3b

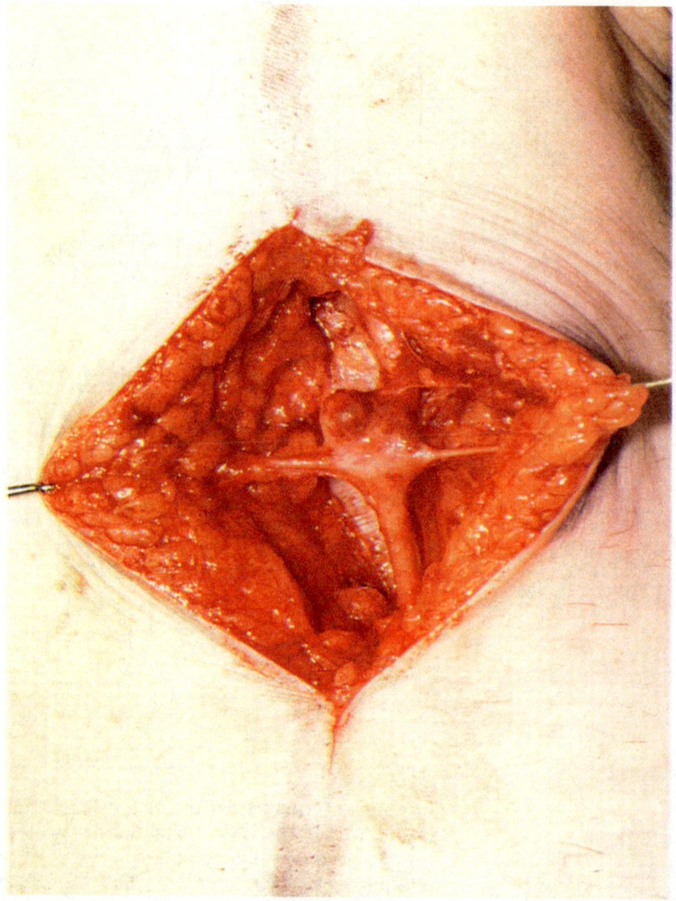

3a and b Typical LSV varicosities. Varicosities on the medial side of the thigh are almost invariably caused by saphenofemoral incompetence i.e. reflux into the long saphenous system from the femoral vein. In the thin patient, on standing, the distended LSV can be readily palpated. In the obese patient it may be well hidden. A 'blow-out' i.e. local ballooning of the LSV at A is very common, particularly in the lower thigh. These blow-outs may mark the sites of incompetent perforators connecting with veins in the subsartorial canal (e.g. the 'mid-Hunter blow-out'), but more often they merely mark the points of entry of distended tributaries which run in a more superficial plane. This dissection shows a 'blow-out' where the LSV is joined by one large and two small tributaries. Varicosities draining the lateral side of the calf and thigh commonly cross above and below the knee to join the LSV. These need to be distinguished from veins draining into the short saphenous vein (SSV).

4 Thigh varicosities. When varicosities are present on the medial side of the thigh, saphenofemoral incompetence is likely to be present. It is a great mistake for the surgeon to ligate only the thigh varicosity without also carrying out saphenofemoral ligation.

4

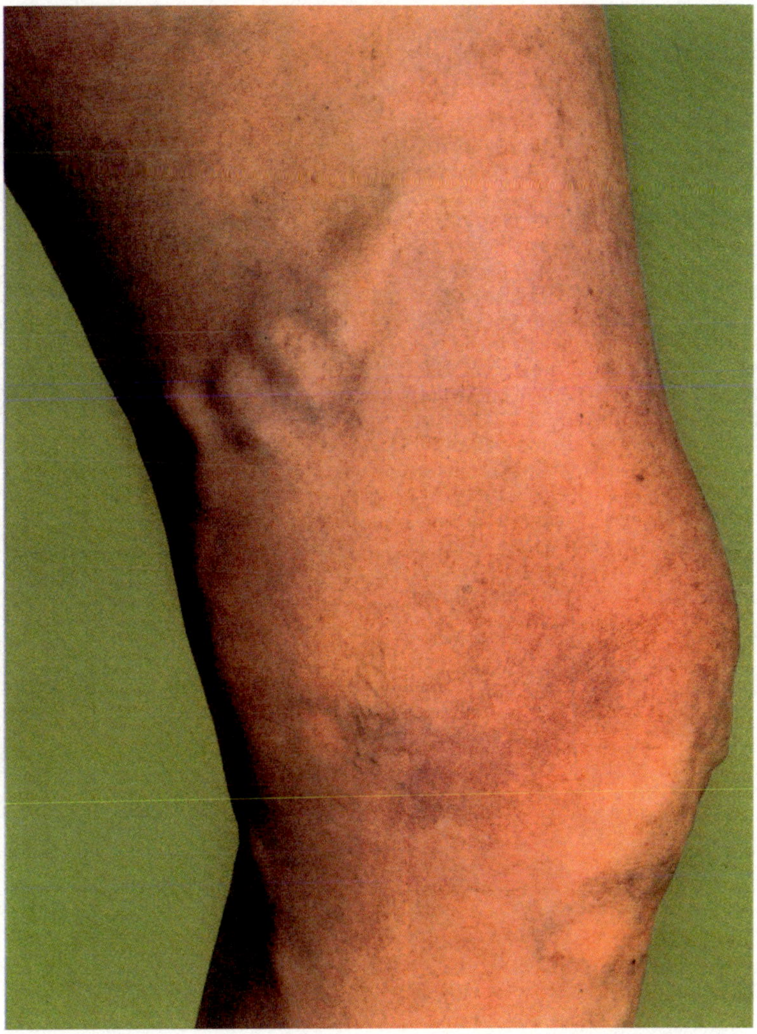

The short saphenous vein

5a, b and c The short saphenous vein (SSV). The SSV begins behind the lateral malleolus by confluence of lateral foot veins. It ascends the median line of the calf posteriorly to end by joining the popliteal vein behind the knee joint. In the lower half of the calf the SSV is associated closely with the sural nerve. Its relation to the deep fascia is variable, usually lying external to it until it reaches the lower border of the popliteal fossa, but in some cases piercing it at mid-calf. The point of entry into the deep veins is also variable and, as indicated by the dotted lines, it may drain into the long saphenous system instead of the popliteal. Often there is also a connection with the long saphenous system at mid-calf level. Varicosities which overlie the SSV do not necessarily drain into it. Varicosities overlying the upper end of the SSV more commonly drain into the LSV, as do those in the upper half of the lateral aspect of the calf. Varicosities on the lateral side of the lower calf frequently drain into the SSV.

A number of perforators are frequently found on the lateral side of the calf. They are smaller than those on the medial side and do not have the same propensity to cause skin changes.

5a

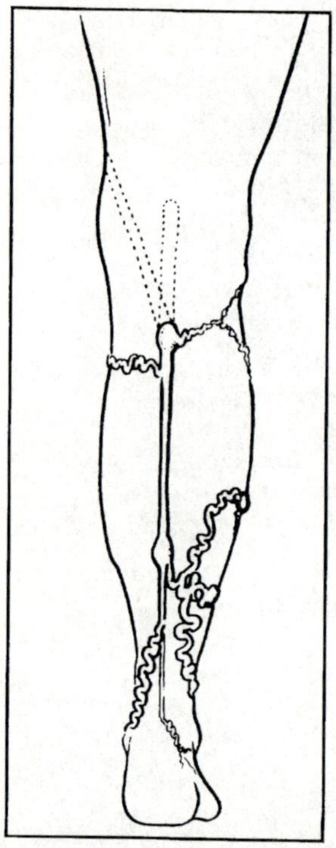

5b

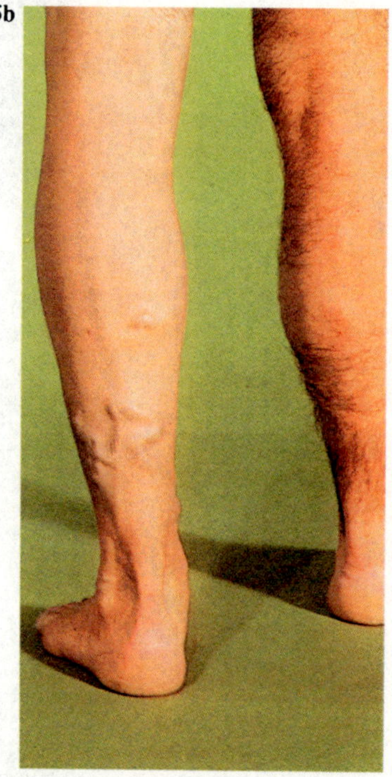

5c

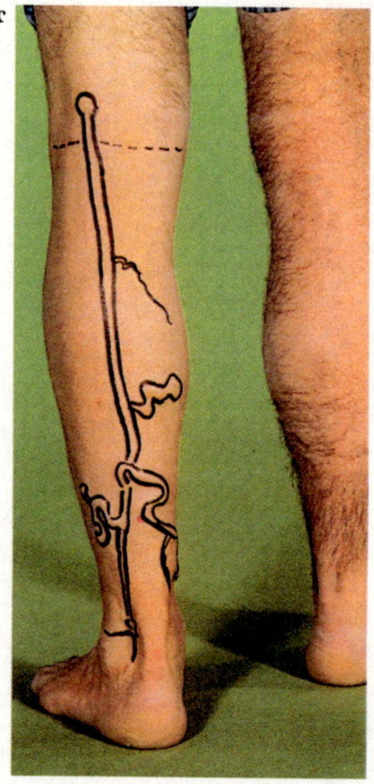

6 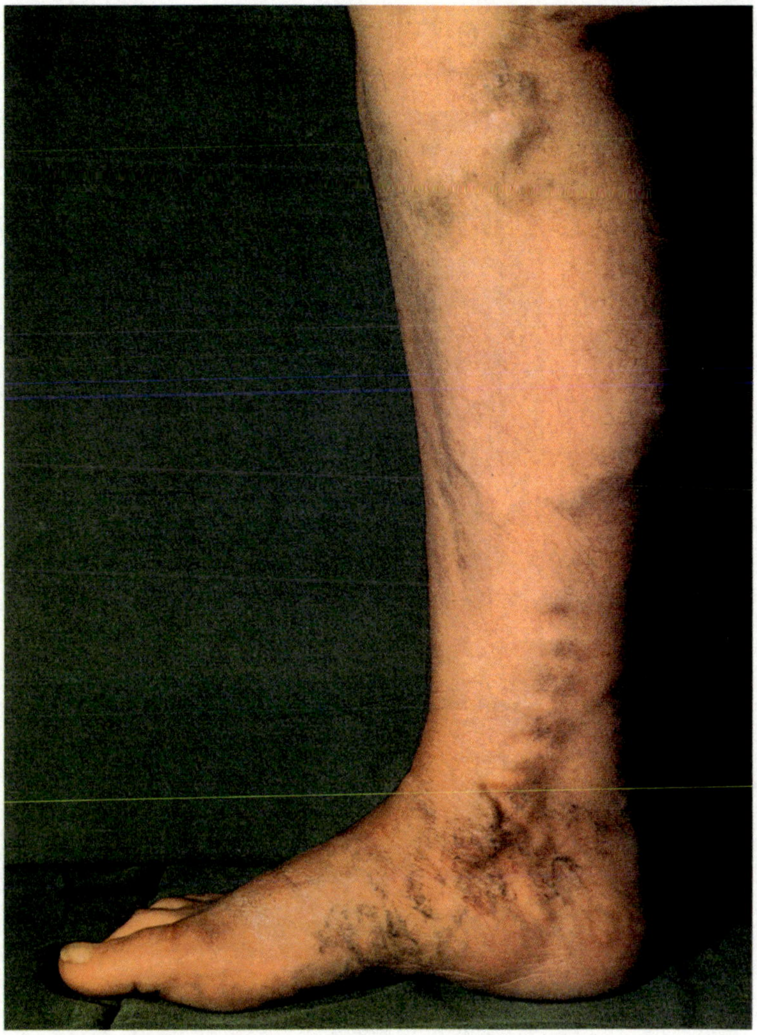

6 Perforator incompetence. Perforating veins at the medial border of soleus, which drain blood inwards from the superficial to the deep intramuscular veins are very constant. If there is a typical venous ulcer present, then it may be assumed that an incompetent perforator lies at its upper end, even although, because of tissue induration, it may not be readily palpable. Similarly, a retromalleolar 'flare' of multiple small subcutaneous or intradermal veins extending down to the sole of the foot is a reliable sign that there is an incompetent perforator at its apex.

Preoperative examination

7

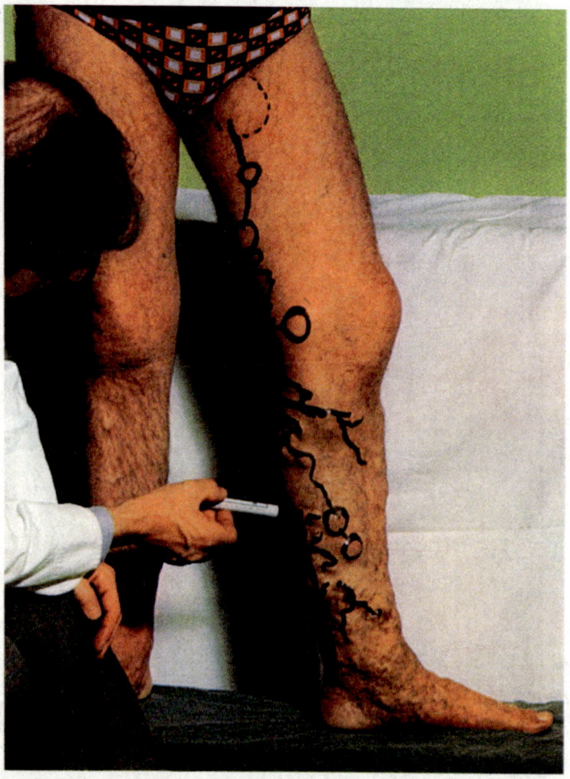

7 Preoperative examination is carried out in good light in a warm room. The patient stands for several minutes on a cloth-covered elevated surface. The surgeon should be seated comfortably, so that he may take ample time to assess and mark the leg.

8

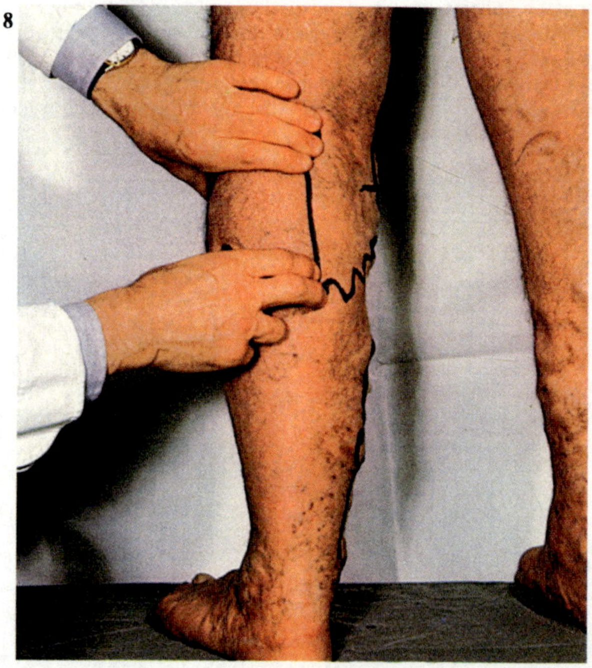

8 Percussion and examination of the short saphenous vein (SSV). Percussion along the line of a distended vein helps to map out the anatomy. Here, the SSV is being examined. The patient stands with his weight evenly distributed and the knee of the affected leg slightly flexed. The surgeon percusses a varix with one hand while the other palpates for the impulse over the upper end of the SSV. An incompetent SSV can usually be felt tense and distended in the popliteal fossa. If in doubt, check with the Doppler.

Tourniquet tests and ultrasound

9

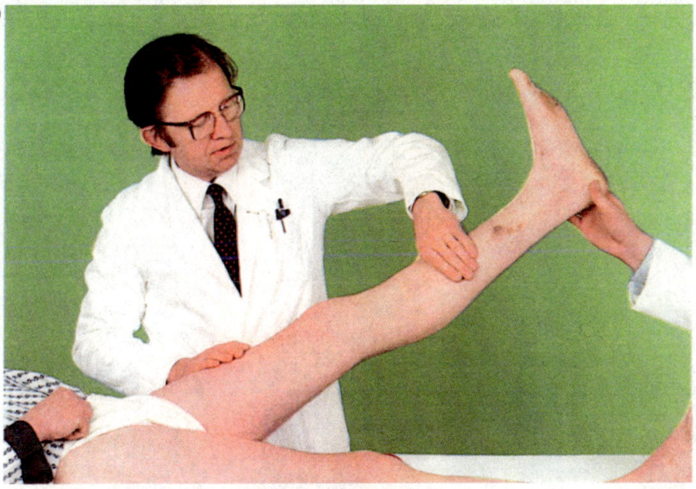

10

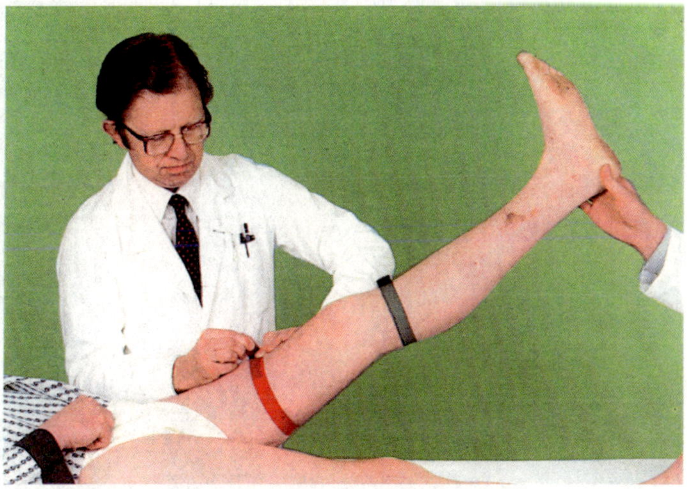

9 Tourniquet test: 1 Elevation of the leg. The tourniquet test is a valuable method of determining levels of incompetence. The patient lies supine. The leg is elevated and the superficial veins emptied.

10 Tourniquet test: 2 Application of tourniquets. The test may be carried out with a single rubber tourniquet (Trendelenberg) or with multiple tourniquets. They are applied with sufficient tension to occlude the superficial veins without occluding the deep arteries or veins. Some surgeons prefer to compress the veins with their fingers rather than with tourniquets.

11

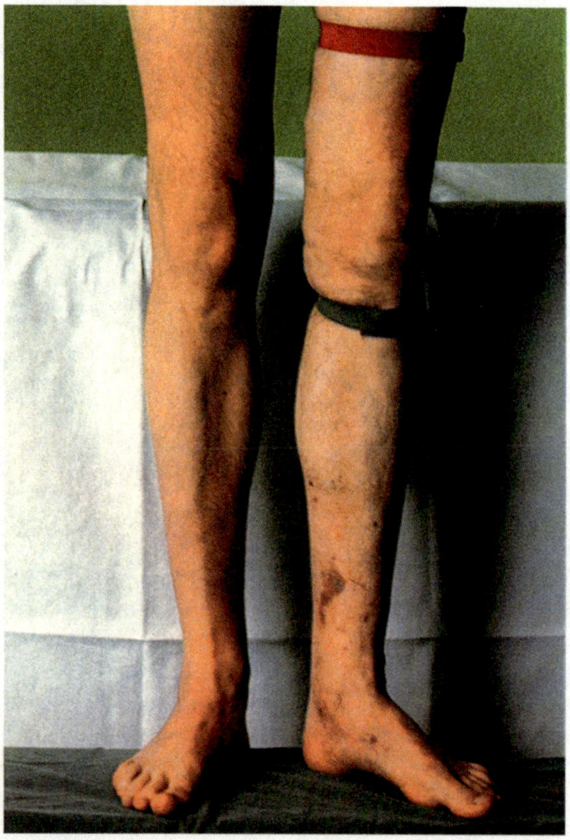

11 Tourniquet test: 3 Thigh perforator incompetence. The leg is then re-examined with the patient standing. Here it can be seen that the varicosities between the tourniquets are distended, indicating an incompetent perforator at that level, while those in the calf are not.

12

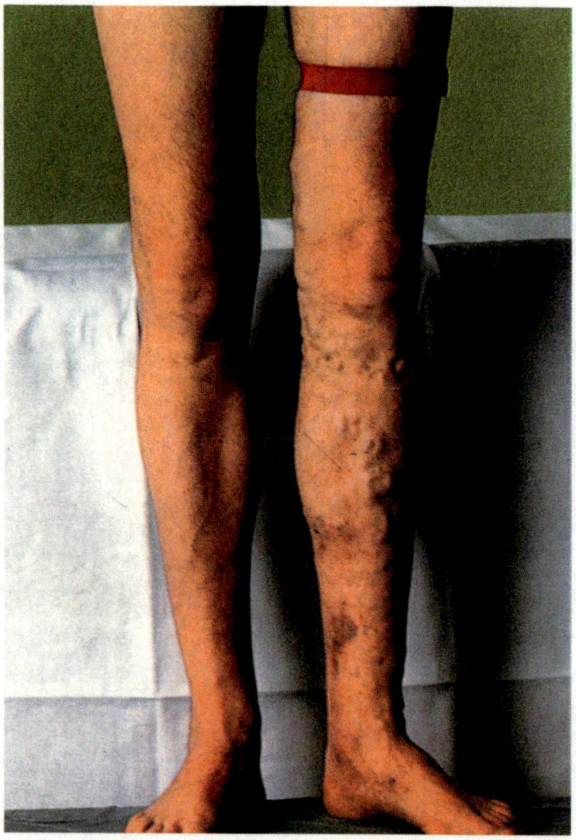

12 Tourniquet test: 4 Removal of tourniquet. Removal of the lower tourniquet shows the calf varicosities filling from a higher level.

13

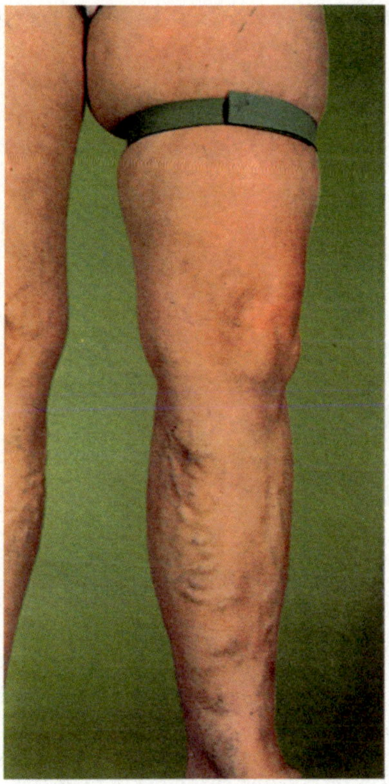

14

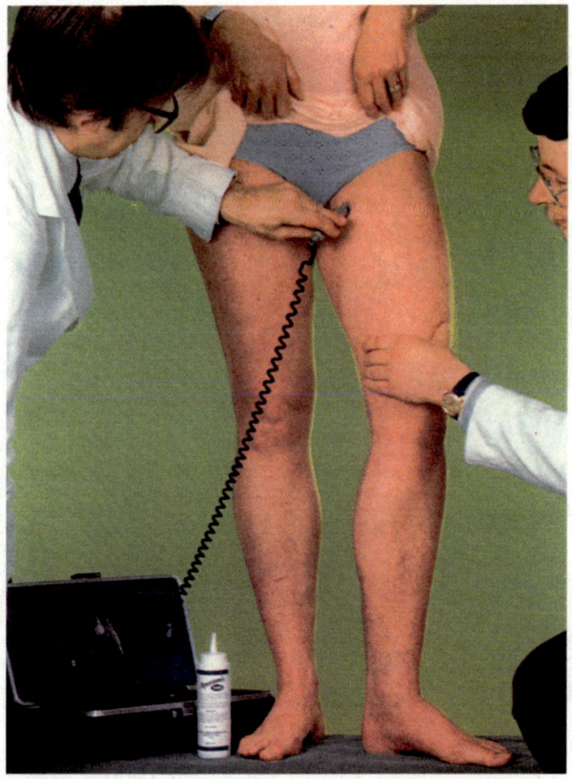

13 Tourniquet test: 5 Calf perforator incompetence. In this patient the calf varicosities are not controlled by the tourniquet, because they are filling by way of incompetent calf perforator(s). The test can be repeated with tourniquets at different levels further to define sites of incompetence.

14 Ultrasound. The Doppler ultrasound machine is a relatively inexpensive portable device which can be a useful adjunct to physical examination, especially in the obese patient. Here the surgeon is listening for reflux in the upper LSV. An augmented signal is elicited by manual compression below the probe. On sudden release of the compression, if the valve immediately above the probe is incompetent, a reflux signal can be heard. If the valve is competent, there is no signal on release of compression. With the knee slightly flexed the SSV can be tested, as can perfector incompetence, with the aid of tourniquets.

15

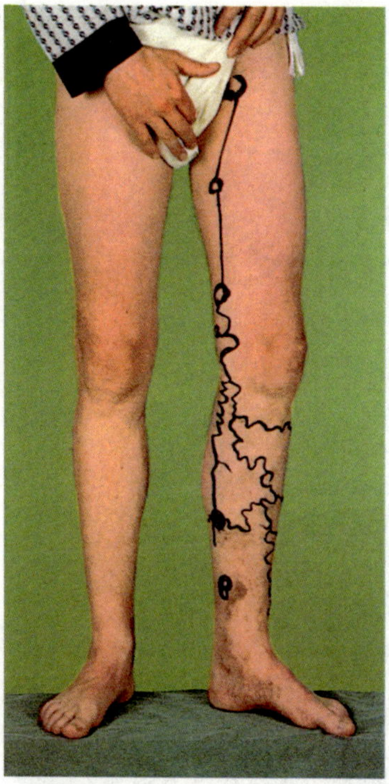

16a

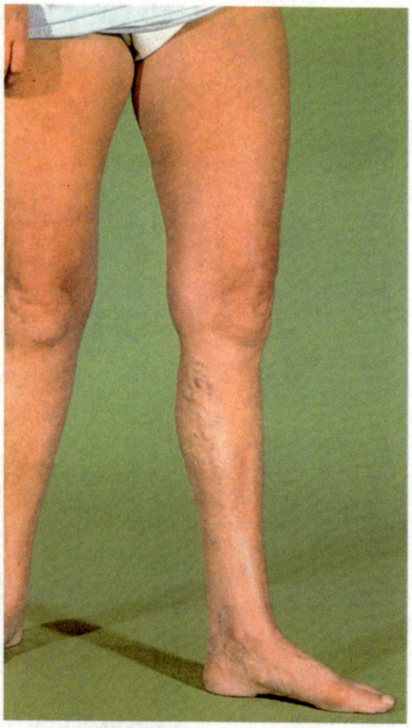

16b

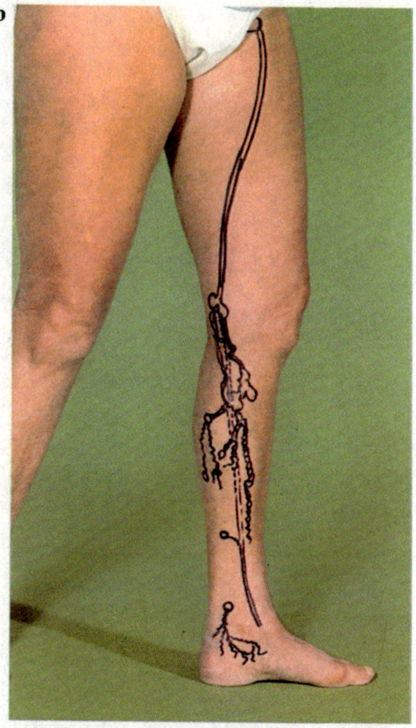

15 The leg is marked. An indelible felt-tipped marker is used to mark the leg, and the incompetent pathways are mapped out. Circles indicate 'blow-outs' at junctions or incompetent perforators. Some examples of common patterns of varicosities are shown in the following figures.

16a and b Long saphenous incompetence. This patient shows large varicosities on the medial side of the calf. Although the LSV is not visible he has obvious incompetence of the long saphenous system. Note the retromalleolar flare (see **6**).

17

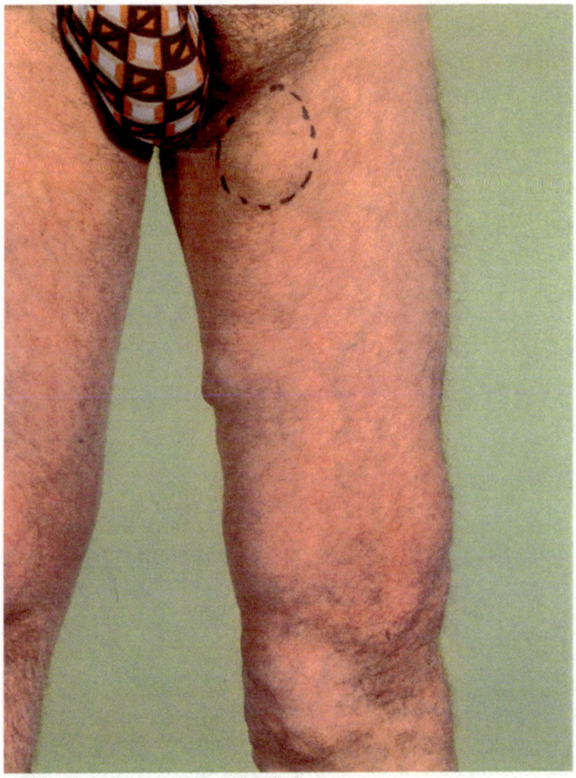

17 Saphenar varix. The saphenar varix, here outlined with a dotted black line, is one of the differential diagnoses of a lump in the groin. Like an inguinal hernia it will manifest a cough impulse. The swelling of a saphenar varix disappears when the patient lies down and the leg is elevated. A saphenar varix is always associated with a distended distal long saphenous system.

18

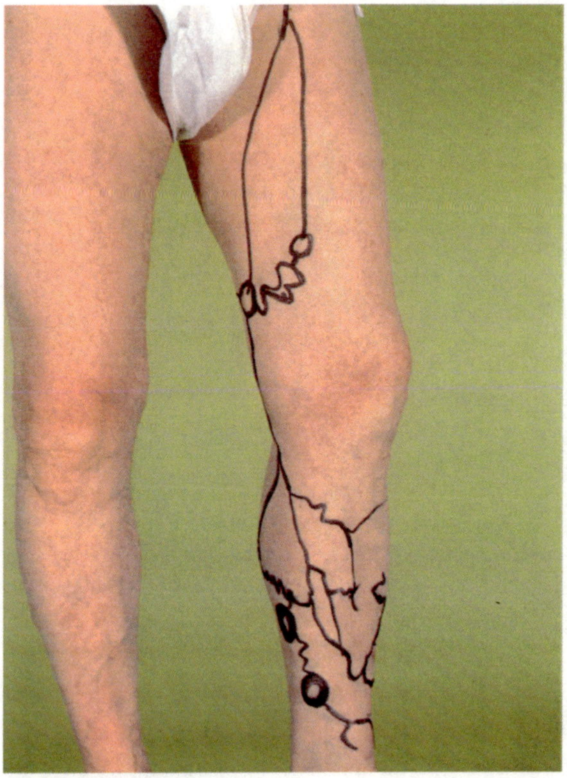

18 Abnormal tributaries at the groin. This patient was found to have two large channels draining up to the groin. The medial one, more deeply placed (and therefore easily overlooked), was the true long saphenous vein (LSV). The other was an abnormal anterolateral tributary (see **41**).

19

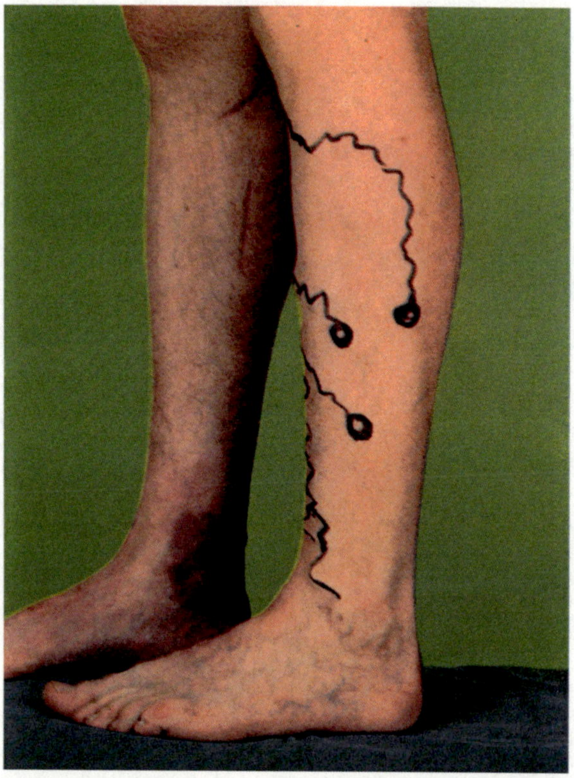

20

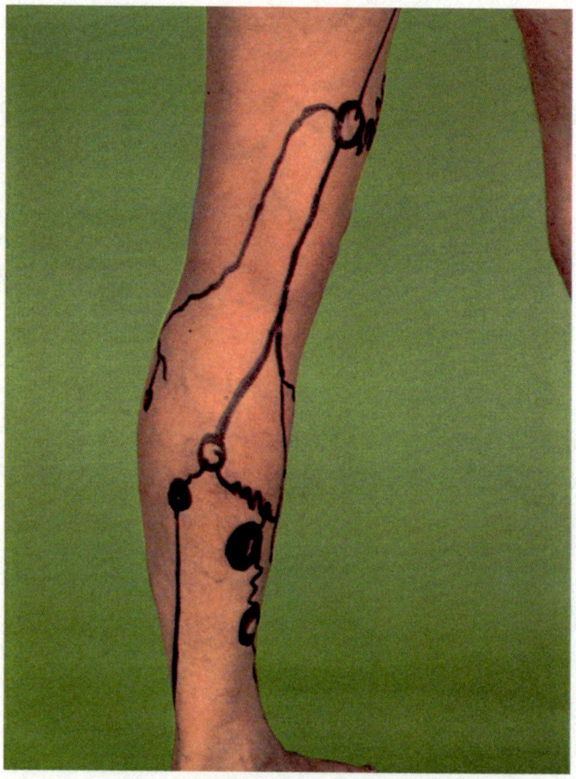

19 Lateral perforators. Varicosities on the lateral side of the calf frequently end at small perforators. Unless they are large, have associated skin changes, or the patient wishes them to be removed for cosmetic reasons, it may be satisfactory to leave them intact, provided that incompetence at a higher level has been treated.

20 Connection between long and short saphenous systems. In this patient the lower half of the SSV was distended below a connection with an incompetent long saphenous system in mid-calf. This is a common anatomical pattern, which has to be distinguished from saphenopopliteal incompetence.

21 Low calf perforator incompetence. This patient has a 'flare' of multiple small superficial varicosities, beginning above the ankle and extending down over the medial side of the foot. This pattern is characteristic of one or more large incompetent perforators on the medial side of the 'gaiter' area of the calf.

21

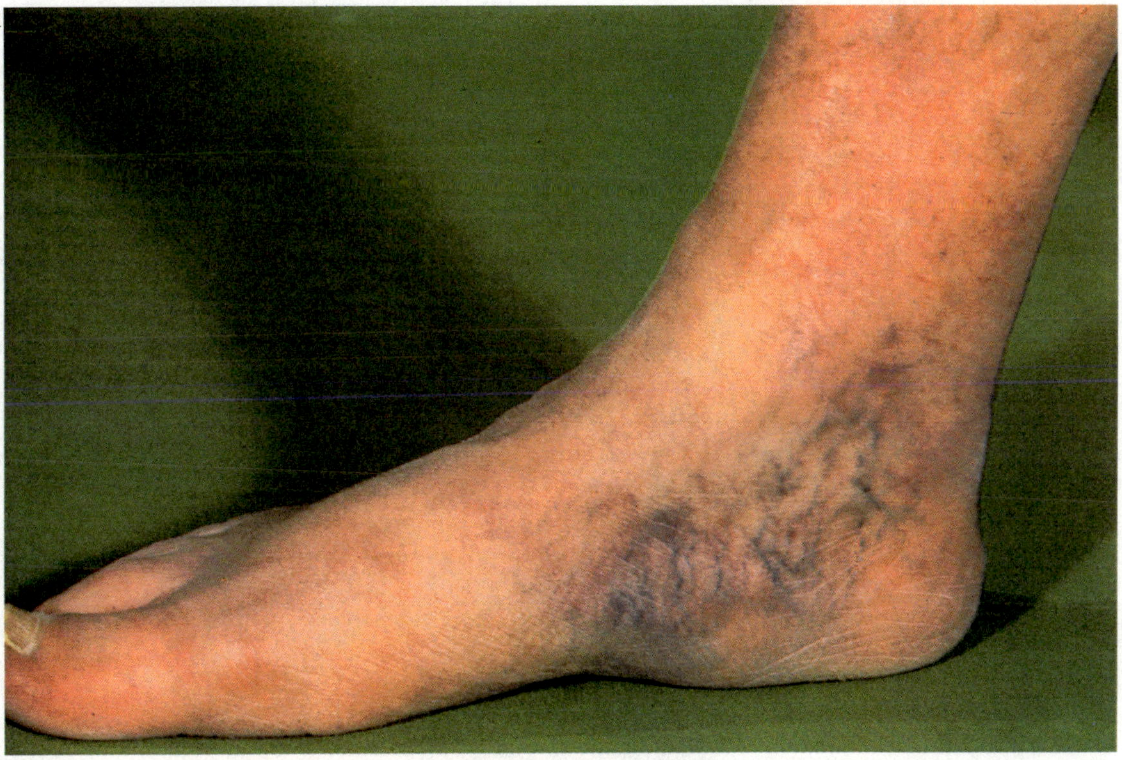

22

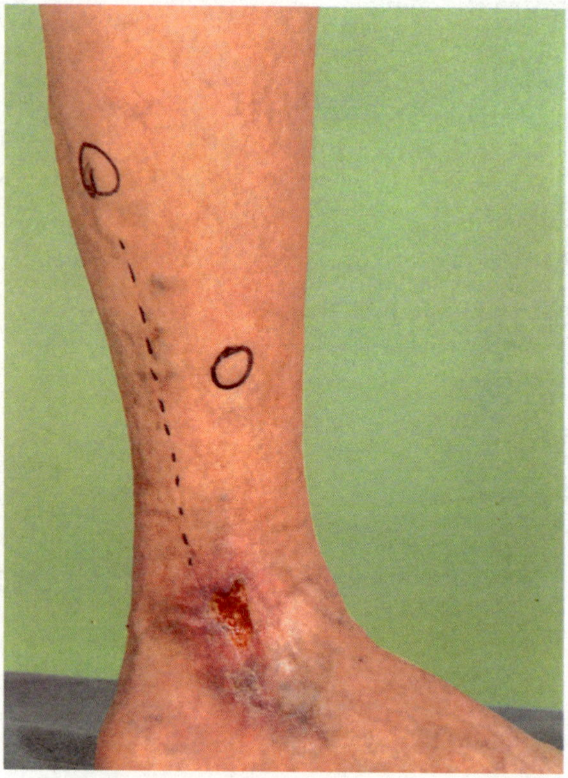

23

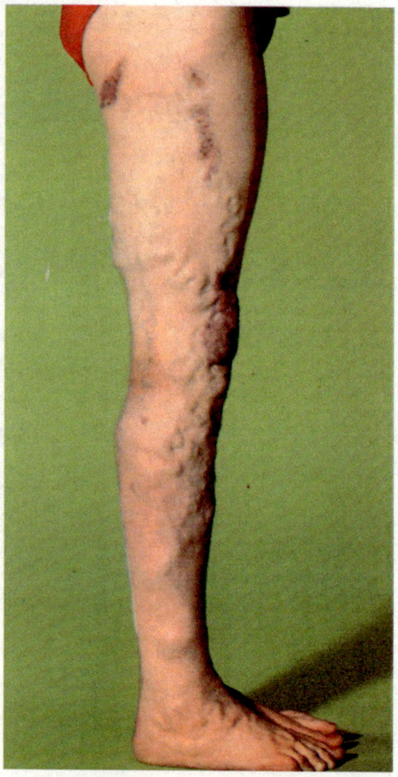

22 Recurrent varicosities with ulcer. The dotted line marks the scar of an extensive previous incision, the operation record stating that subfascial ligation was performed, despite which there are evidently large incompetent perforators still present. Recanalisation is possible, but it is more likely that the perforators were not recognised and dealt with at the previous operation.

23 Posterolateral varicosities in the thigh may be a sign of congenital venous anomaly such as the Klippel Trenaunay syndrome, or as in this case of arterio-venous fistula.

Position during operation and skin preparation

24

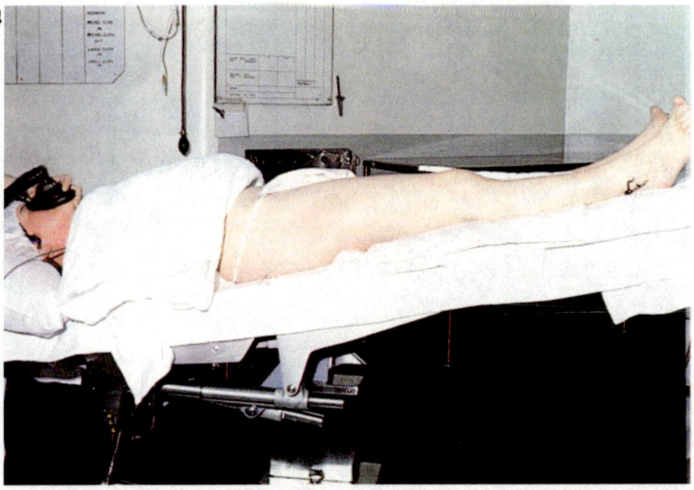

25

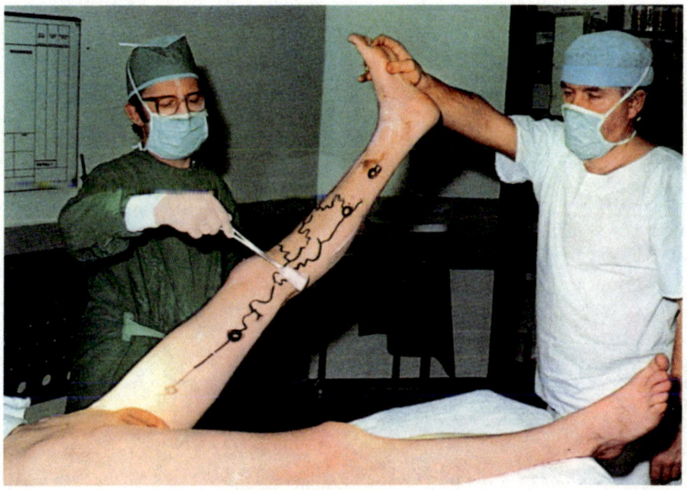

26

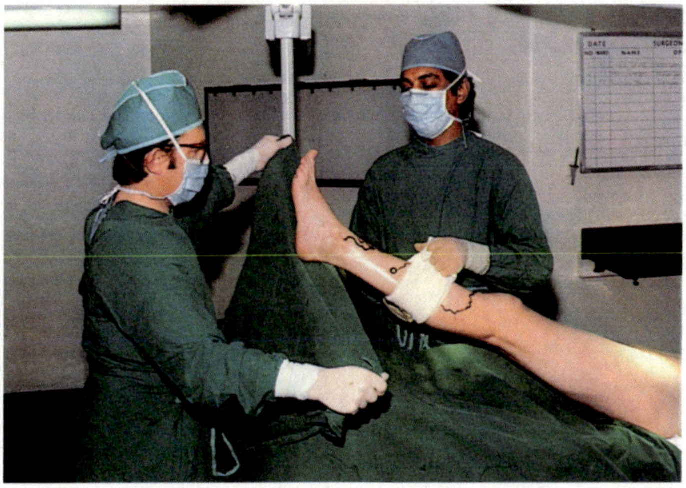

24 The position during operation. Elevation of the legs at an angle of about 10 degrees during the operation avoids venous distension and minimises bleeding. Should heavy bleeding be encountered during the saphenofemoral dissection, it can be controlled readily by increasing the tilt of the table and applying local pressure – *not by grasping blindly with artery forceps*. With the help of suction and pressure above and below, the bleeding point is then dealt with by ligature or suture as required.

25 Skin preparation. The entire leg, the lower abdomen, the groins, and genitalia are painted with antiseptic.

26 Draping the foot 1. The assistant supports the leg while the foot is draped. The towel is folded to the shape of a triangle.

27

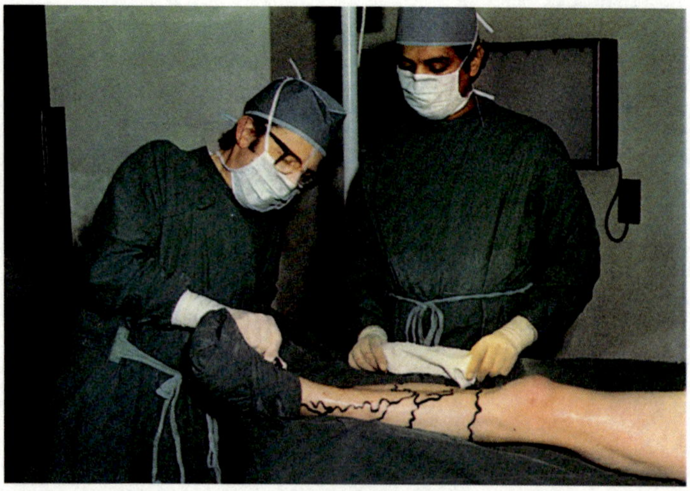

28

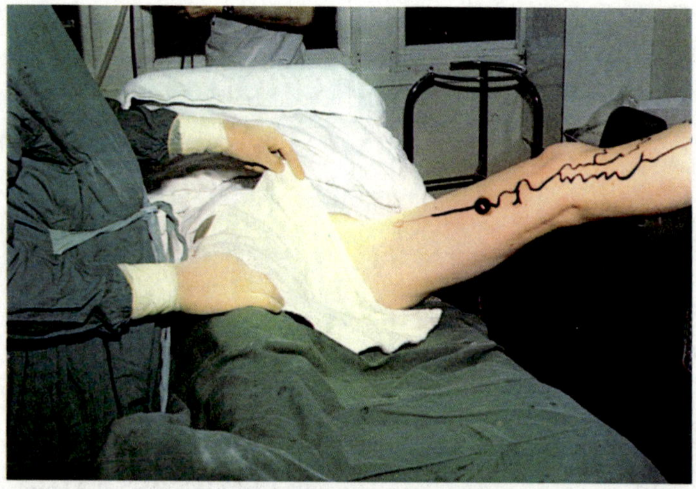

29

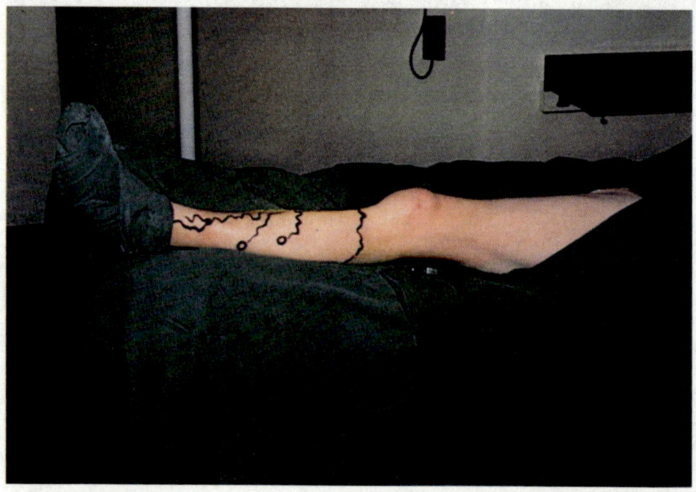

27 Draping the foot 2. The towel is firmly folded around the foot and ankle and secured.

28 Draping the groin. Care is taken to seal off the genitalia and perineum with a single layer of Terry towel, which is tucked under the buttock.

29 Access. Draped in this way, the leg can be moved freely into a variety of positions to facilitate access at various points.

The Trendelenberg procedure

30
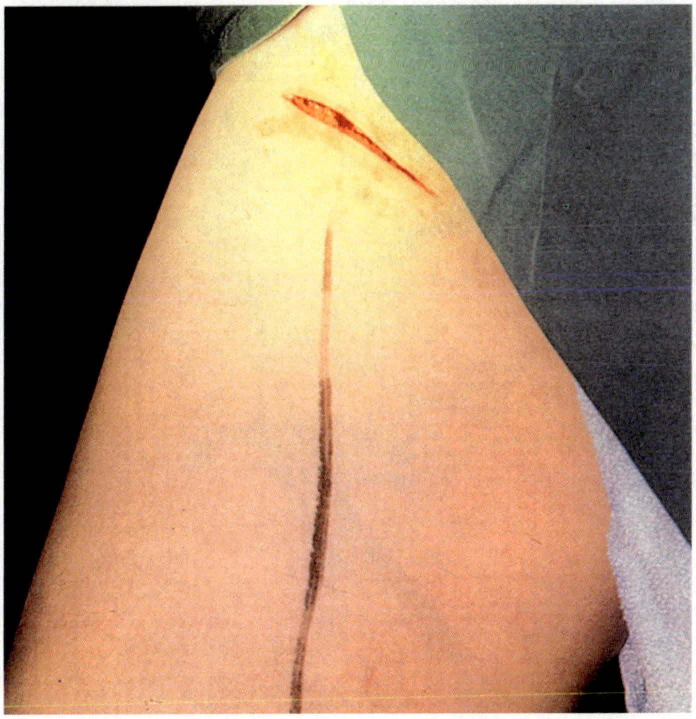

31
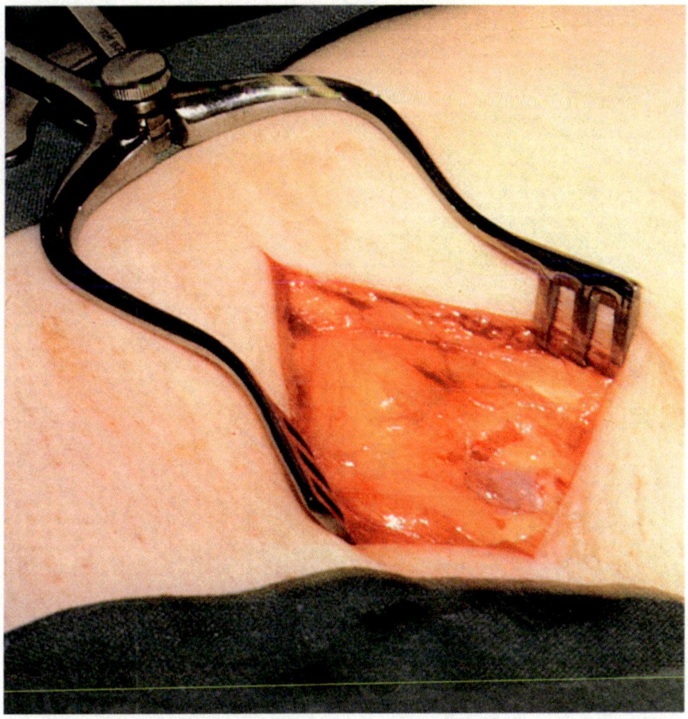

30 The Trendelenberg procedure 1. A 6cm to 8cm incision is centred on a point 3cm to 4cm below and lateral to the pubic tubercle. This is the point at which the LSV pierces the cribiform fascia to enter the femoral vein.

31 Locating the long saphenous vein (LSV). The incision is deepened to the membranous layer of the superficial fascia. A self-retaining retractor is inserted. The upper end of the LSV can usually be seen through the membranous layer, but if not, readily comes into view as the dissection is deepened.

32

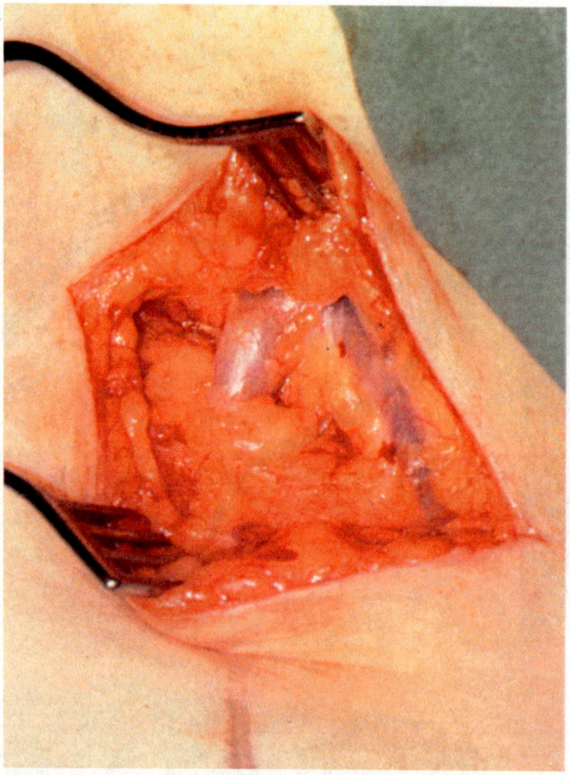

33

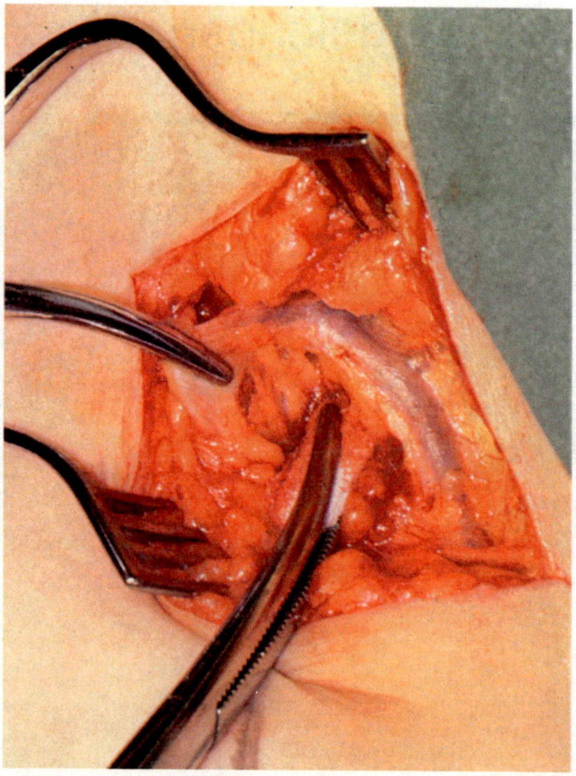

32 Anatomical variants. Be prepared for anomalies such as this large high tributary (see **18**).

33 Exposure of the long saphenous vein (LSV). The venous anatomy is defined with a dissecting pledglet.

34

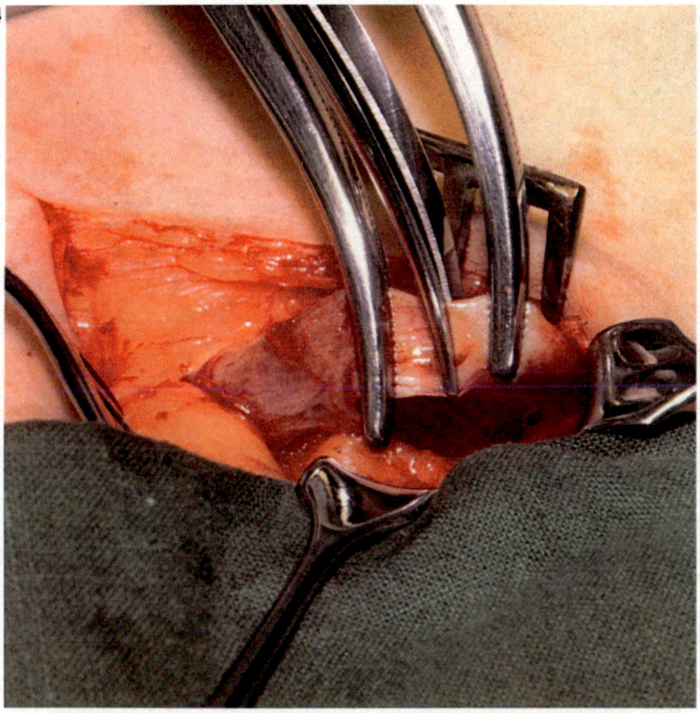

35

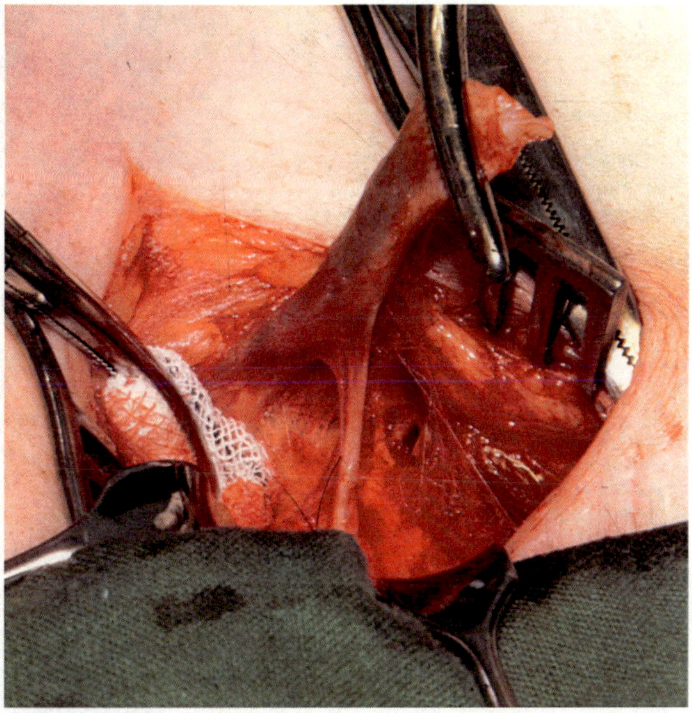

34 Mobilisation of the long saphenous vein (LSV). The dissection is deepened and the vein mobilised. In thin individuals the femoral artery and vein can be situated quite close to the skin surface – therefore a good deal of caution should be exercised to ensure that neither is mistaken for the saphenous vein. *Provided that the surgeon is quite certain that he is dealing with the correct vessel*, it can be picked up and divided between Mayo's artery forceps. This facilitates dissection of the tributaries and display of the saphenofemoral junction.

35 Exposure of the saphenofemoral junction. Elevation and moderate traction of the proximal stump facilitates dissection and displays the tributaries.

Ligation of tributaries

36

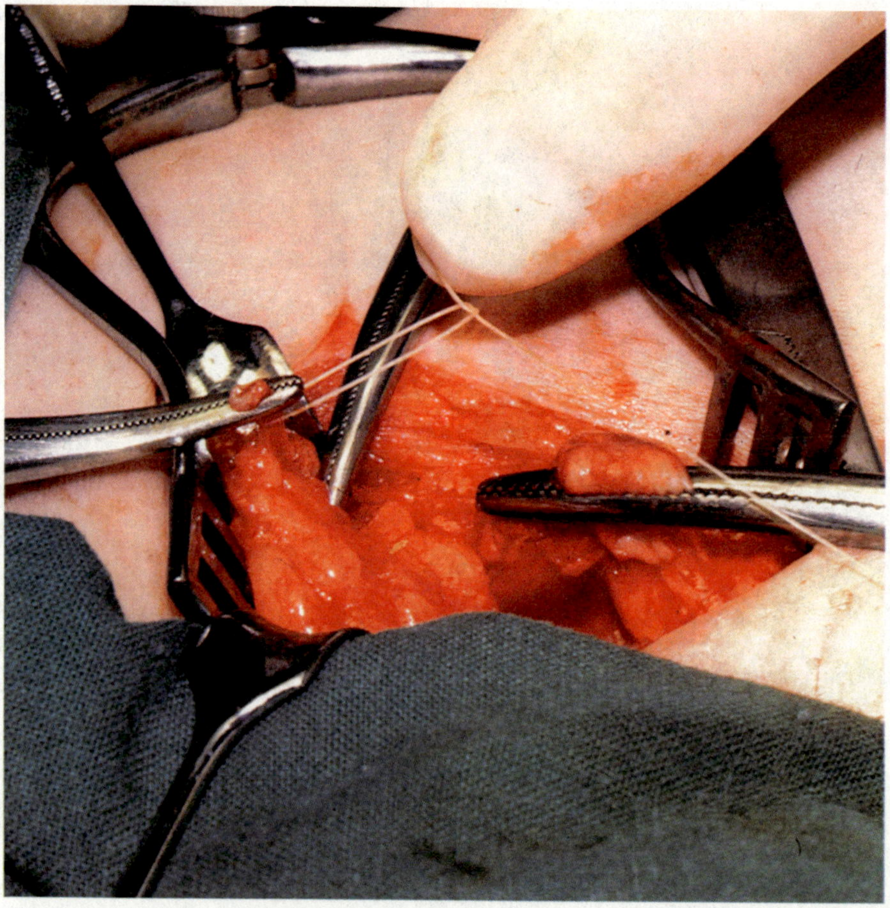

36 Ligation of the tributaries. The tributaries are divided and ligated with 3/0 catgut. Normally there should be at least three: the superficial external pudendal, the superficial circumflex iliac, and the superficial inferior epigastric. The assistant should take care not to lever on the artery forceps while the superficial inferior epigastric vein is being tied – the stump of an avulsed vein may be difficult to find. The superficial external pudenal artery crosses the upper end of the LSV immediately below the saphenofemoral junction. It may be left intact or ligated between silk ligatures to facilitate the mobilisation of the vein.

37 **Recognition of the saphenofemoral junction.** The LSV pierces the cribiform fascia to enter the common femoral vein. As the stump of the LSV is elevated by traction on Mayo's forceps, the junction can usually be identified as a white line (arrowed).

37

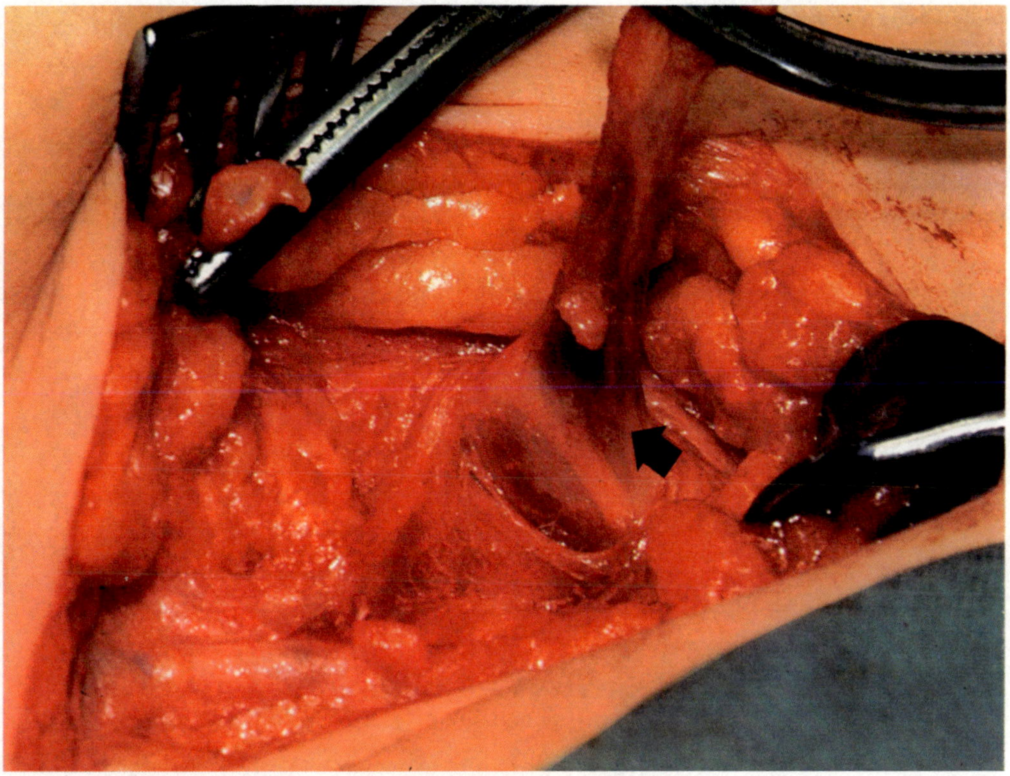

38 Transfixion of the long saphenous vein (LSV). The stump of the LSV is transfixed with a non-absorbable suture (braided nylon in this case) on a round-bodied needle. Although this procedure is often termed 'flush ligation' it is important not to place the transfixion suture too close to the femoral vein because of the risk of constricting it – especially as the femoral vein can readily be tented up by traction on the LSV stump. The transfixion suture is therefore placed 1 cm to 2 cm from the junction.

38

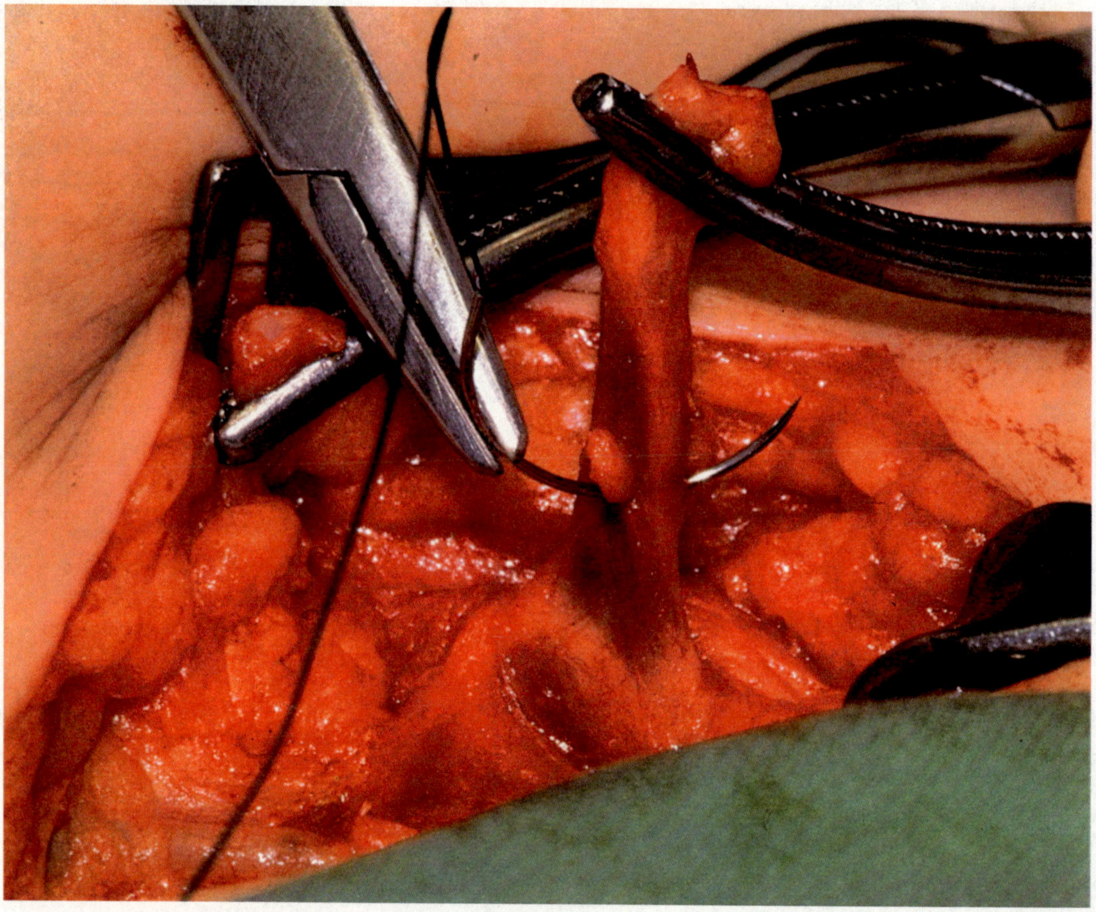

39 The saphenous stump. The ligated vein is trimmed back leaving a generous stump of vessel beyond the ligature, so that there is no risk of the latter slipping off.

39

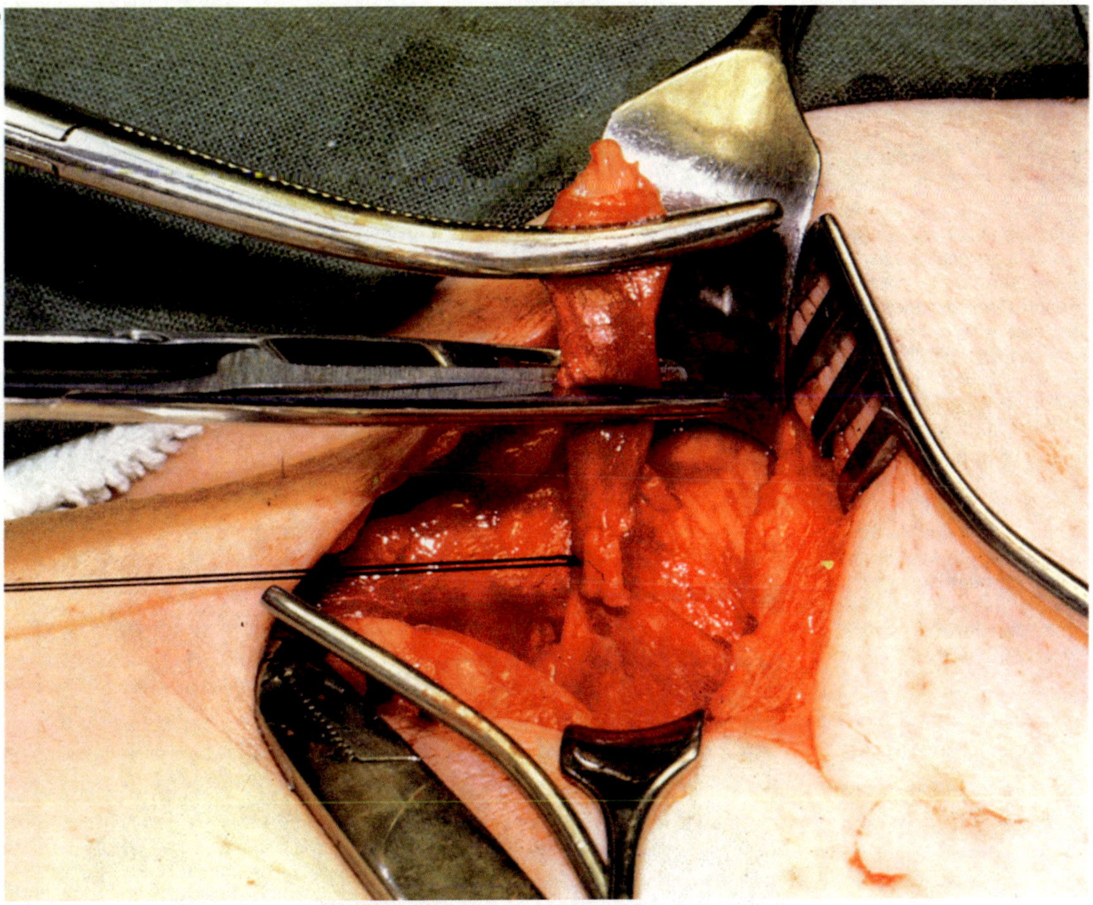

Long saphenous vein tributaries

40 Thigh tributaries. Tributaries of the LSV which join it high in the thigh – notably the postero-medial superficial femoral vein – should be sought through the groin incision. The knee is flexed and the thigh abducted. Traction on the LSV and mobilisation with the finger, as shown, usually allows the medial tributary to come within range of artery forceps. If, as in this case, a tributary is palpable too far down for it to be easily ligated through the groin incision, access may be gained through a small separate incision.

40

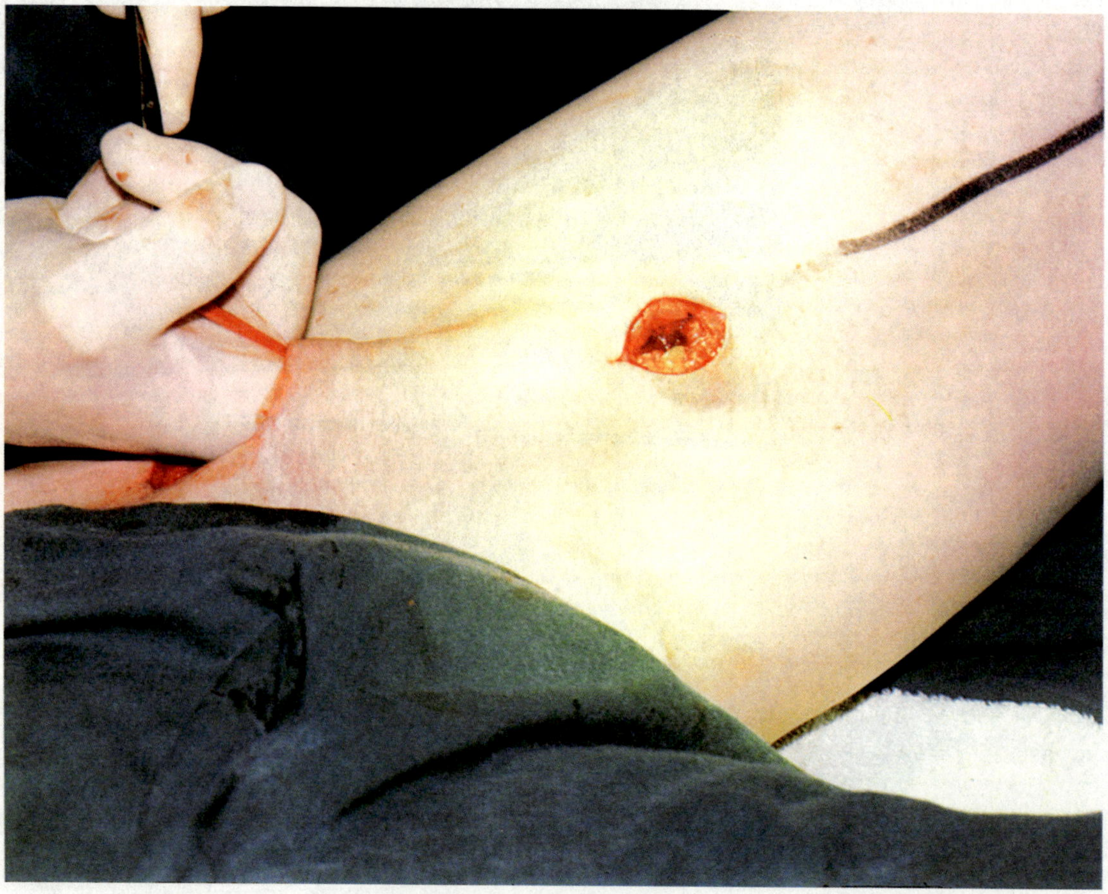

Pitfalls of the Trendelenberg operation

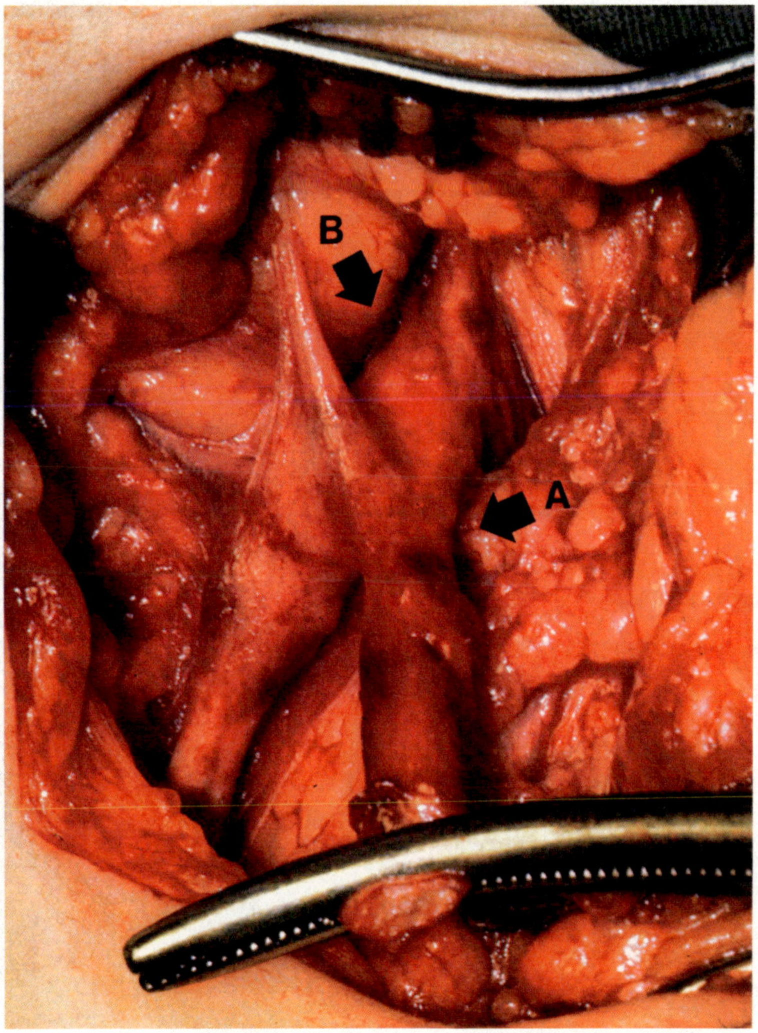

41

41 Trendelenberg operation – pitfalls. As mentioned earlier, anatomical variations are quite common. The tributaries at the saphenofemoral junction are usually three in number; the superficial circumflex iliac; the superficial inferior epigastric and the superficial external pudendal but they may vary in number and position. The posteromedial thigh vein usually joins the LSV about 6cm to 8cm below the saphenofemoral junction, but it may join right at the junction (illustrated here), as may the anterolateral vein of the thigh, and either may be mistaken for the LSV. This is a potential cause of recurrent varicosities. Thus the tributary may be ligated where it joins the LSV (arrowed at A), the surgeon believing that he is carrying out saphenofemoral ligation (arrowed at B). Hence a generous incision (5cm to 7cm) should be made for this operation. Good retraction and thorough dissection are necessary to display the anatomy.

Anatomical variants

42 Anatomical variant. In dealing with abnormal anatomy the minor tributaries are ligated as described earlier. The anatomy is carefully checked to make sure that the femoral artery and vein are at a deeper level. The saphenous vein and the large tributary are divided, held in artery forceps and the saphenofemoral junction defined.

42

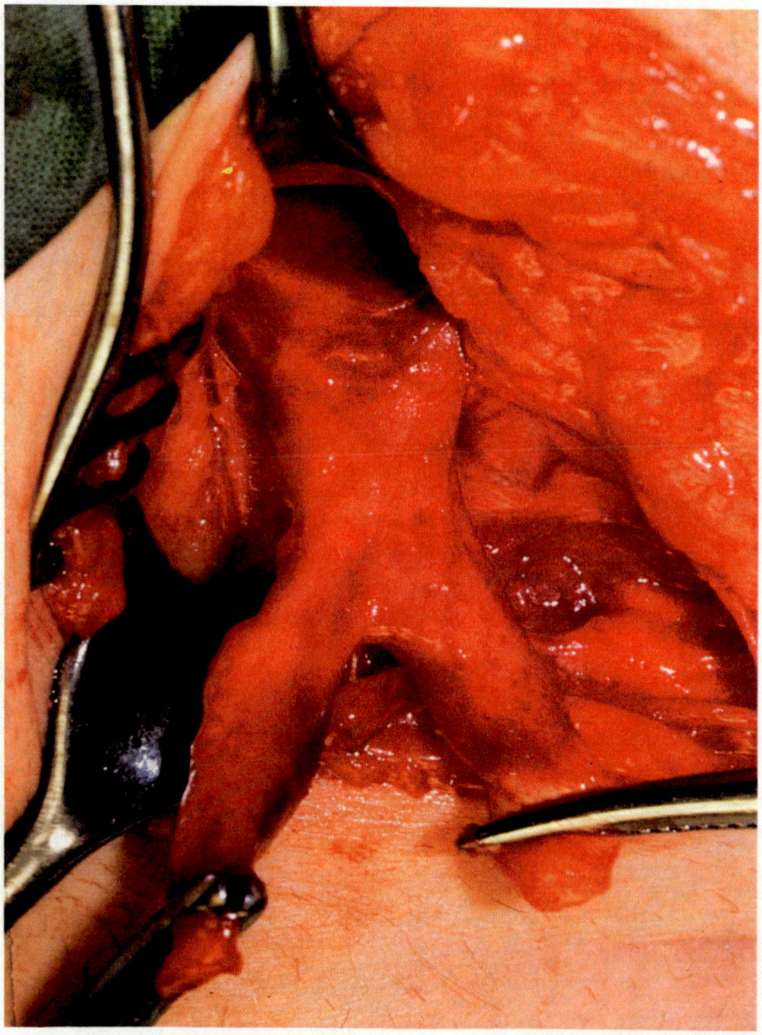

43 **Anatomical variant.** The LSV and the large tributary are separately transfixed and ligated.

43
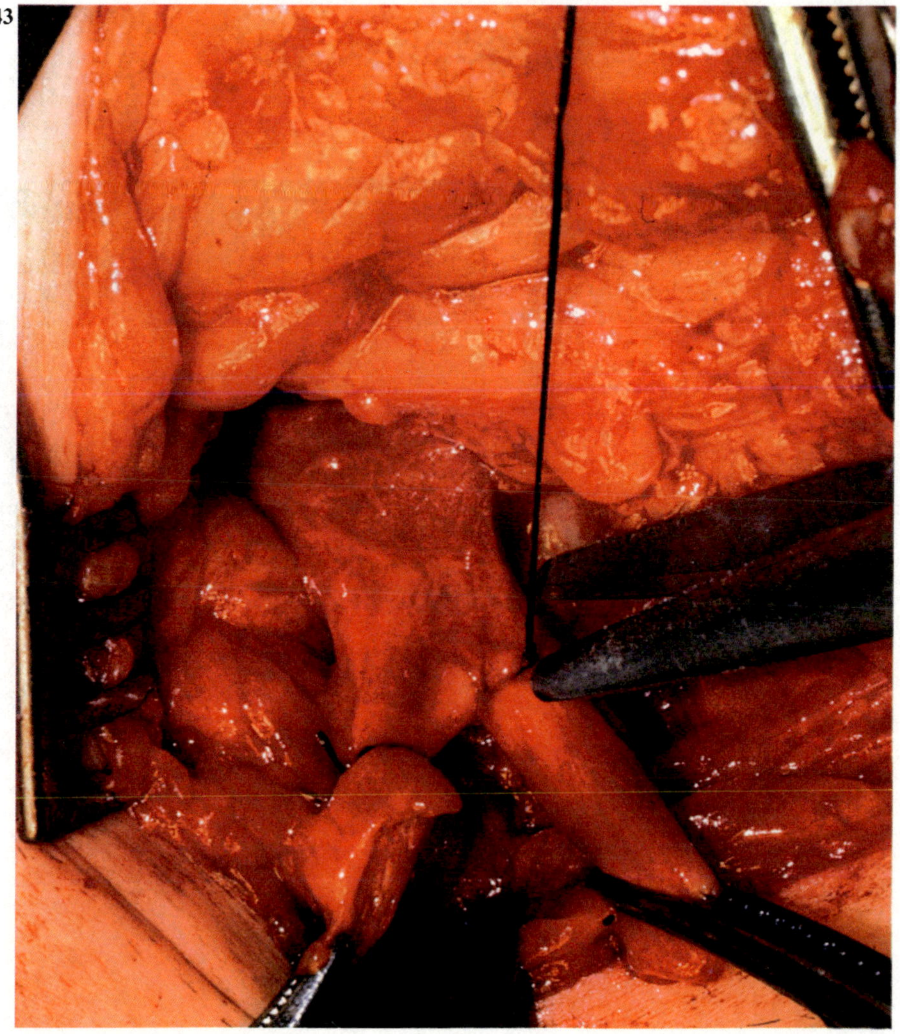

Ligation of short saphenous vein

44 Short saphenous ligation. Most patients with short saphenous incompetence also require surgery to the long saphenous system. If the patient is not obese and has free joint movement, adequate access to the popliteal fossa may be achieved with the patient in the supine position. Otherwise it is necessary to turn the patient prone after the anterior ligations have been carried out. If only short saphenous ligation is required the prone position is preferred. It is particularly important that the anatomy should have been accurately assessed and marked before operation, because the incision of choice is a transverse one. This limits the scope for dissection longitudinally.

44

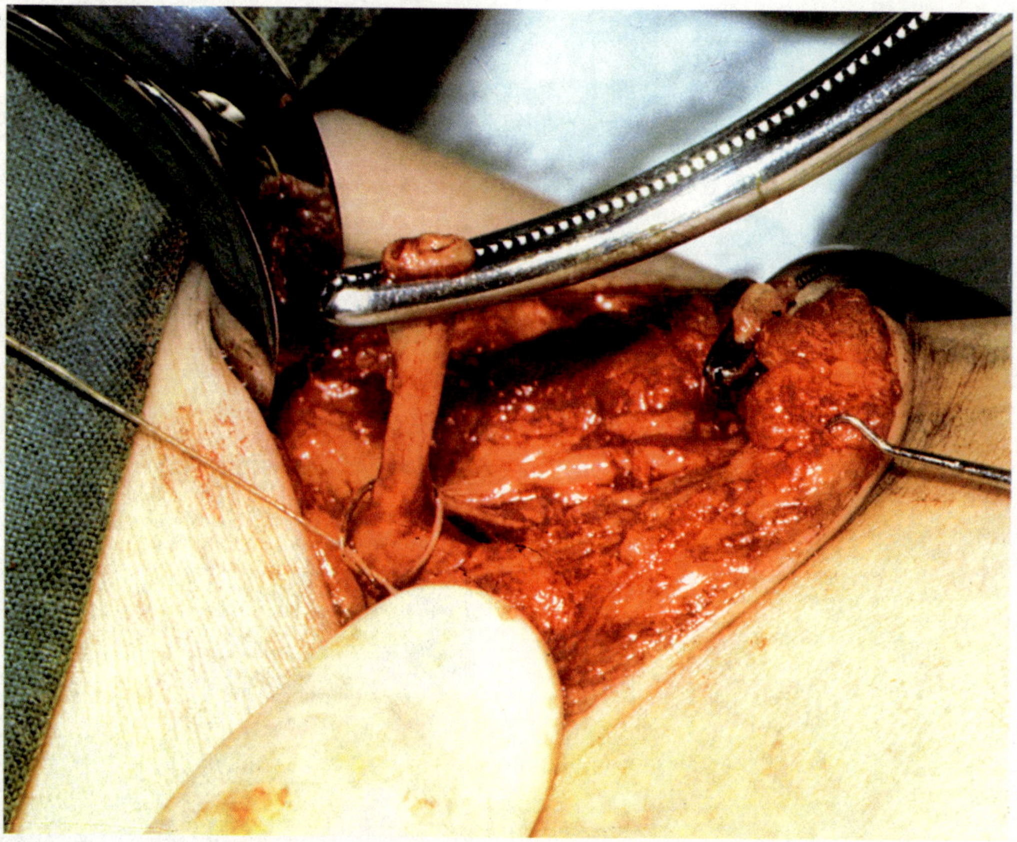

44a

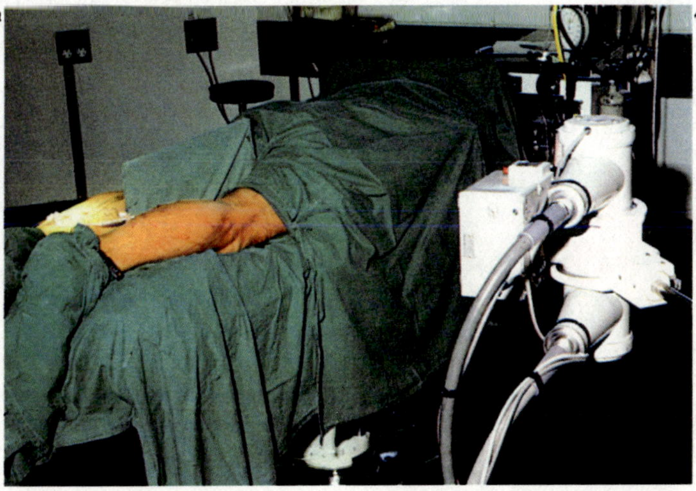

44b

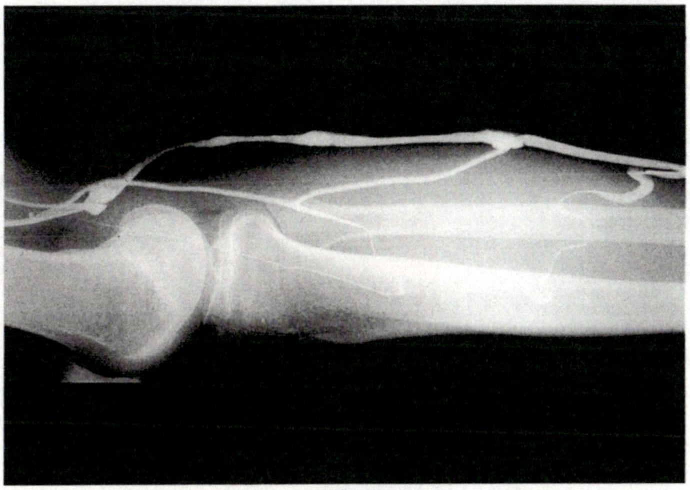

44a and b Phlebography of the short saphenous vein (SSV). If there is doubt about the venous anatomy a preoperative phlebogram is recommended. The short saphenous vein (SSV) is exposed in the lower calf and cannulated. A cassette wrapped in a sterile towel is positioned medial to the knee. 10ml to 20ml of Conray 280, diluted 50 per cent in isotonic saline, or one of the newer non-ionic contrast media is hand injected. A single lateral view is all that is required.

Alternatively the phlebogram can be performed before the leg is painted and draped.

Stripping and removal of vein

45

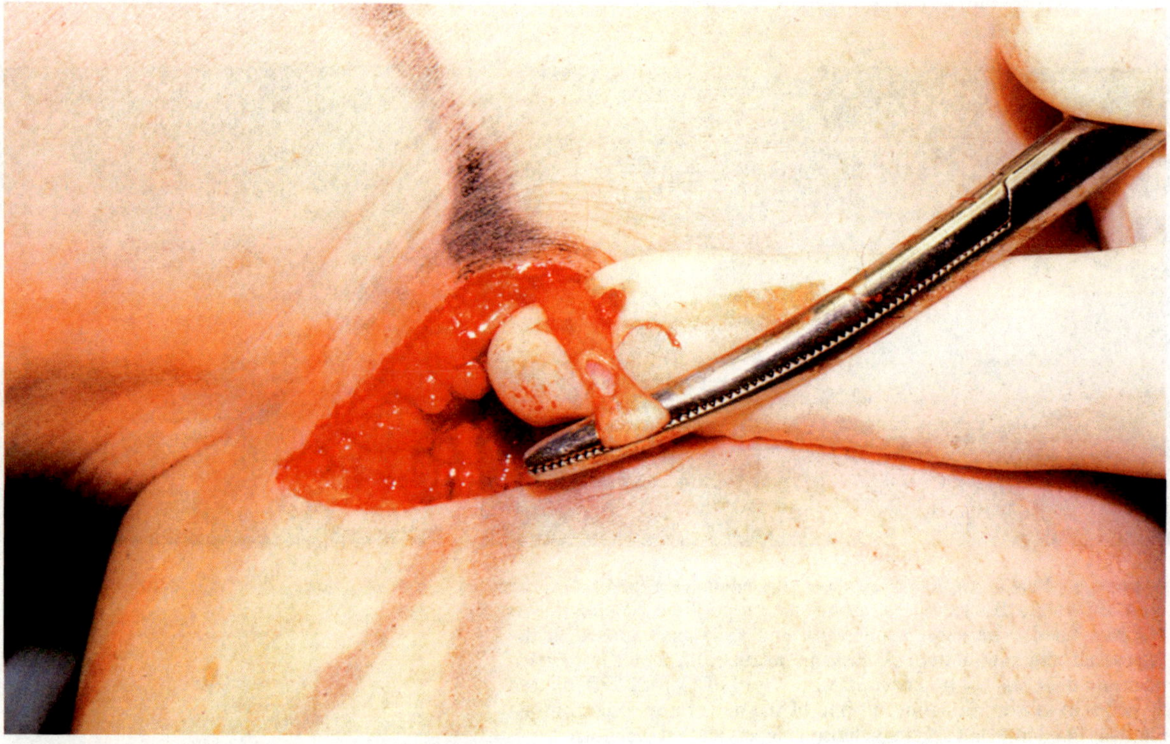

45 Stripping. The upper end of the LSV has been dealt with by the Trendelenberg procedure as described previously, and an artery forceps left on the distal stump. The LSV is exposed through a skin crease incision two fingers breadths below the joint line posteromedial to the knee. It is controlled with an artery forceps distally and incised transversely for insertion of the stripper.

a

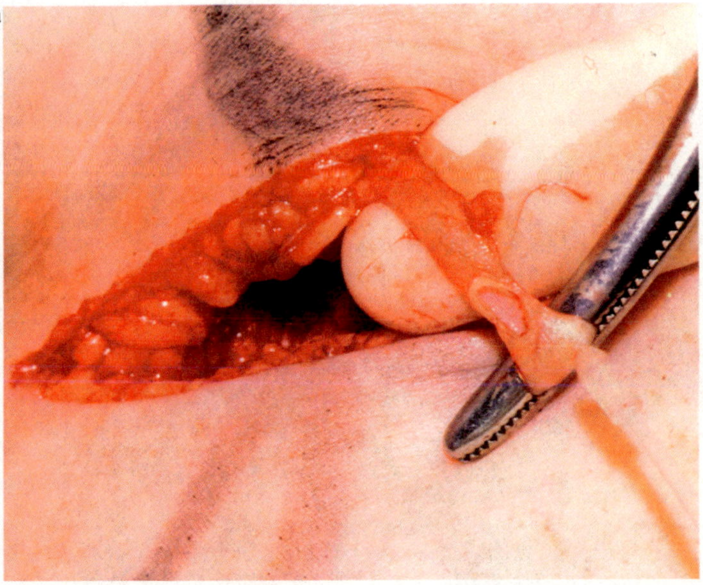

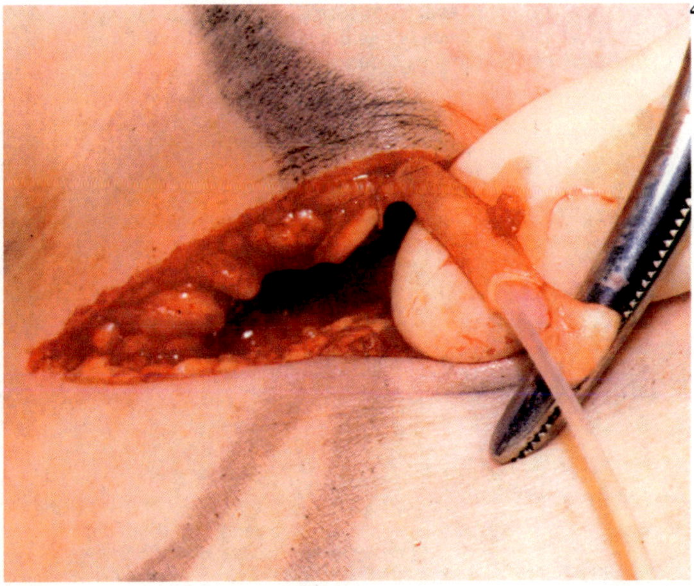

46b

46a and b Insertion of the stripper. The stripper is introduced and passed proximally. Occasionally occlusion of the LSV or sacculation at a junction with a tributary in the thigh prevents passage of the stripper. In such a case the site of obstruction is explored.

47 Securing the lower end. An acorn appropriate to the size of the vein is chosen. A heavy ligature secures the divided vein to the stripper adjacent to the acorn.

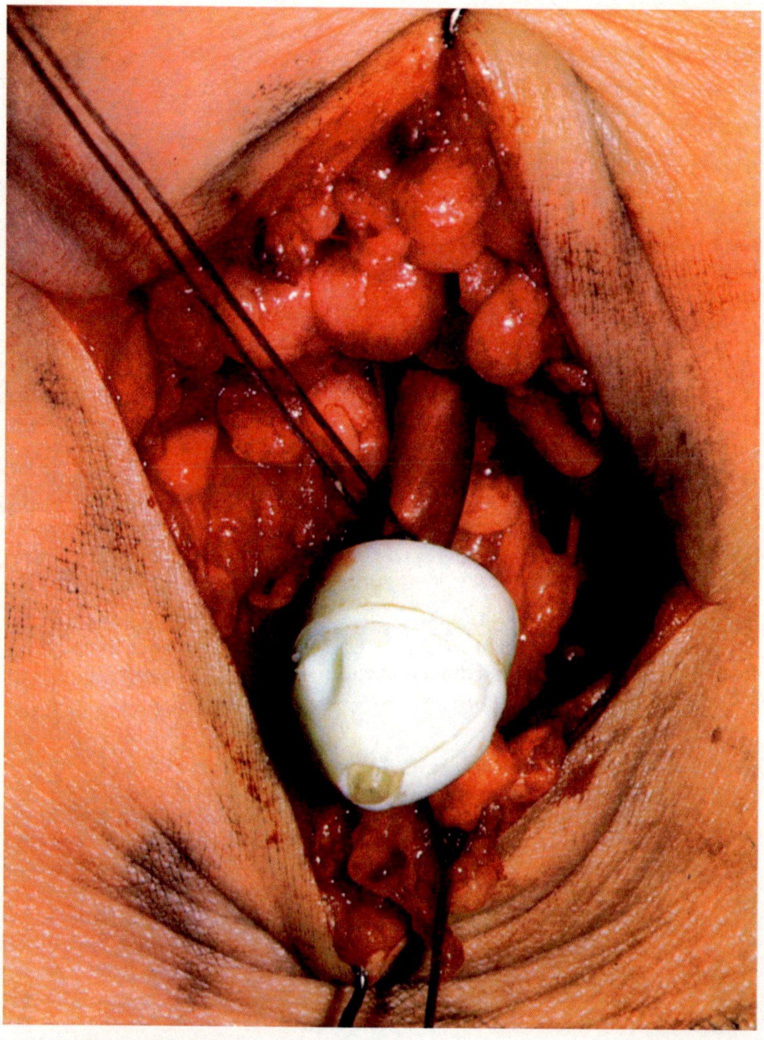

47

48 The stripper is secured at the groin. The distal stump of the LSV at the groin is tied to the stripper. The stripper is left *in situ* until the remainder of the operation, at other sites on the limb, is completed. The upper end of the stripper is brought out through the lateral end of the groin wound which is closed, except that the last skin suture at the lateral end is left untied until the leg has been bandaged and the stripping completed.

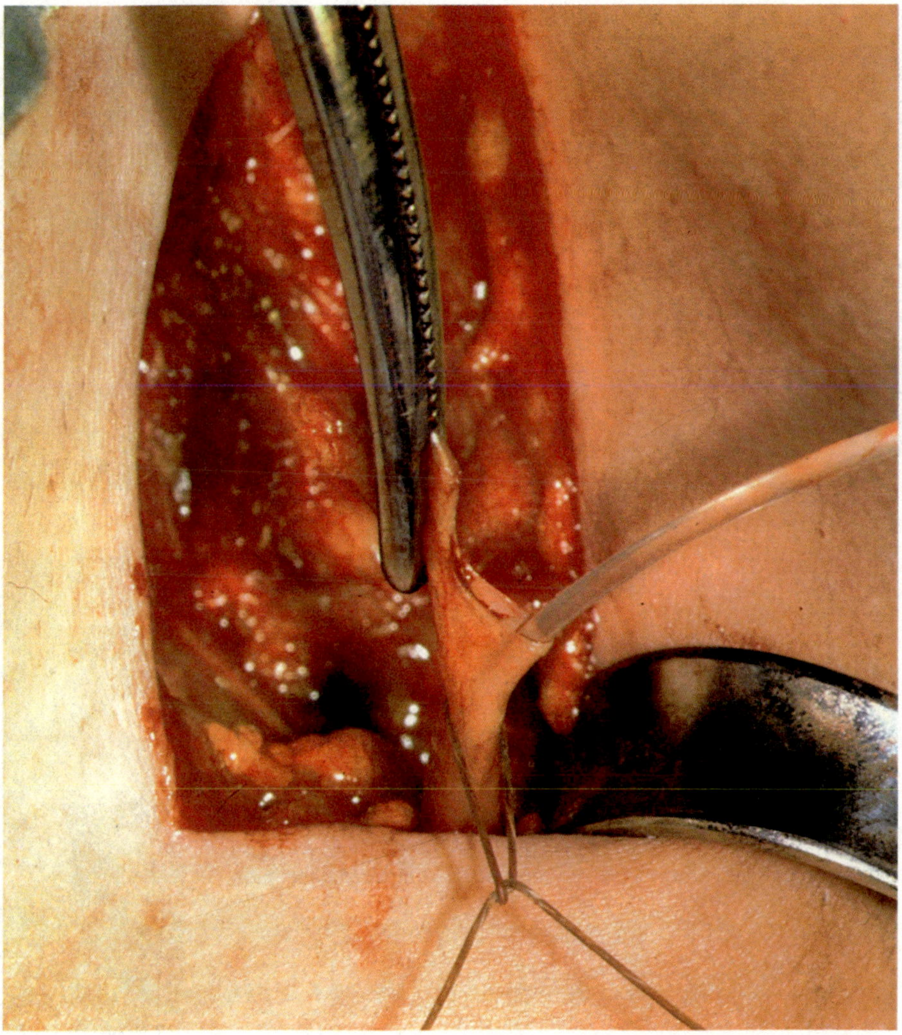

48

49 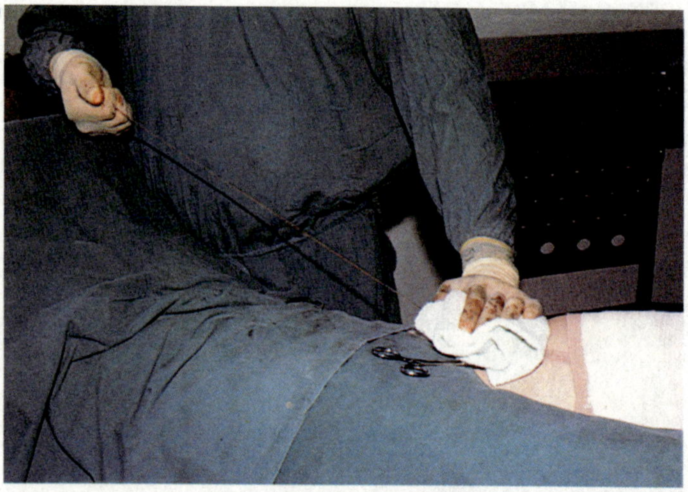

50 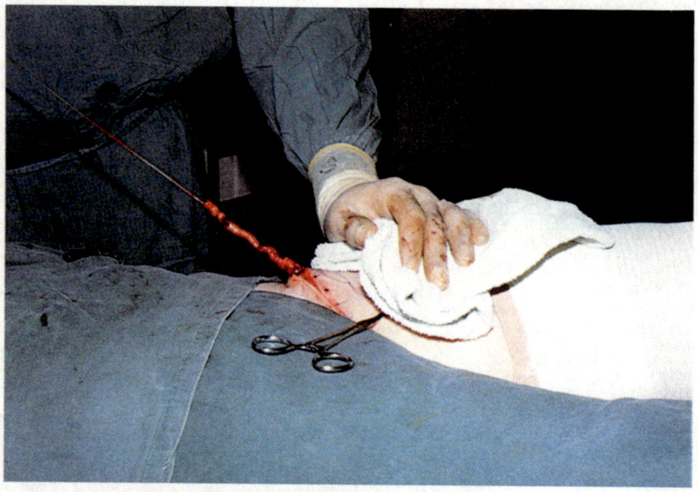

49 Stripping. The leg is dressed and bandaged as described later (see **76** to **80**). The elastic compression having been applied, the LSV is stripped out from knee to groin. Here the surgeon is applying pressure over a folded towel with his left hand, while stripping the vein with his right.

50 Removal of the vein. The 'concertinaed' vein is eased out through the wound. The last untied suture is held on forceps and tied.

51 Completing the closure at the groin. Finally the last suture is tied while the leg is raised to assist haemostasis. If the high thigh tributaries have been properly dealt with, as described in **40**, and the bandaging correctly applied, there should be no haematoma formation. To complete the operation a dressing is applied to the groin wound.

51 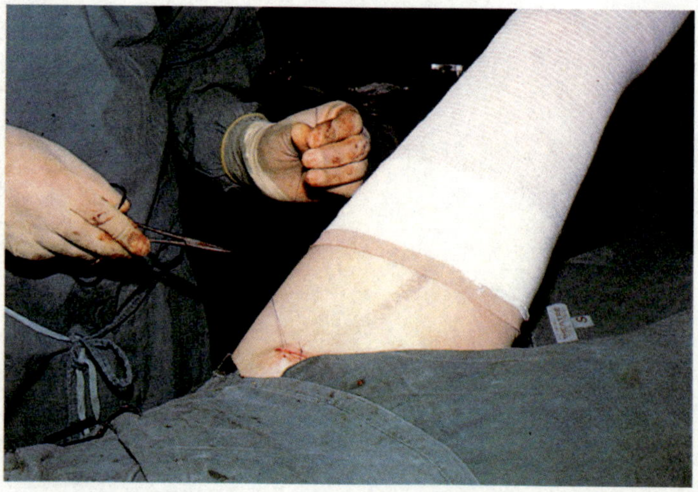

Multiple ligations

52

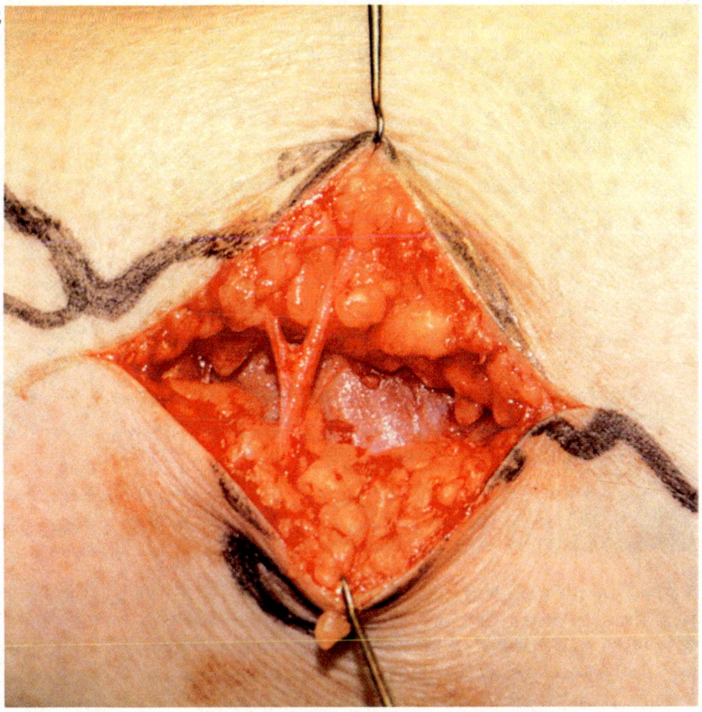

53

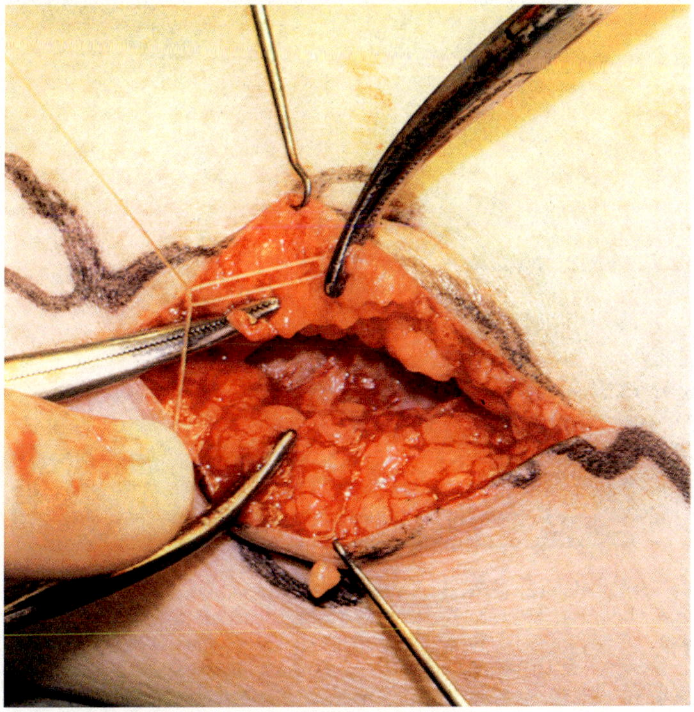

52 Incisions. Longitudinal incisions are the rule except near joints where the incisions are made in skin creases. The wound edges are retracted with skin hooks.

53 Ligations. Veins are divided and ligated, but excessive dissection in the superficial subcutaneous plane is avoided.

54

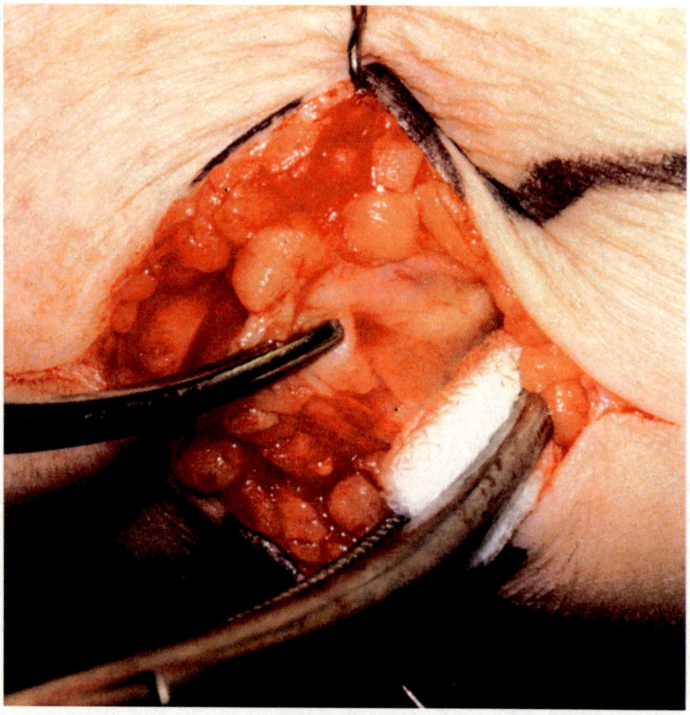

55

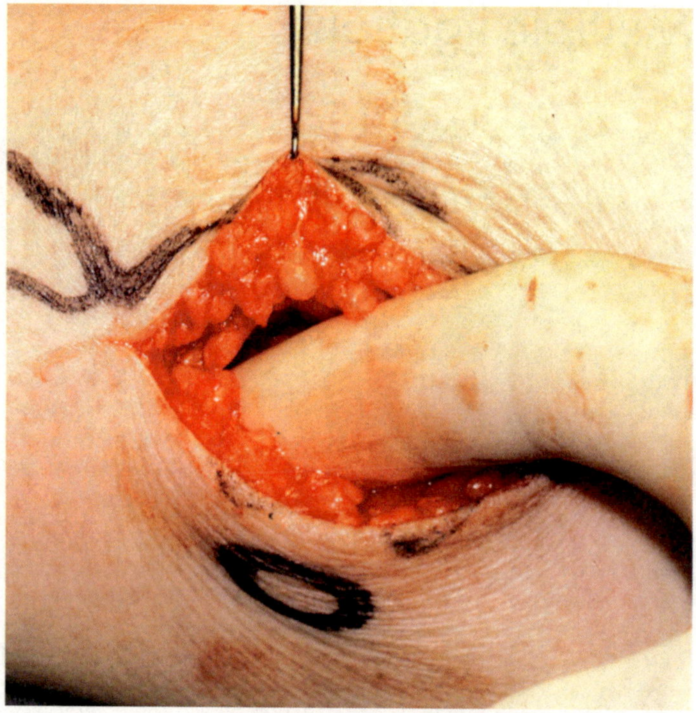

54 Deepening the dissection. With the help of a dissecting pledglet held in a Mayo's artery forceps, the dissection is carried down to the fascia lata.

55 Freeing the tissues at the level of the deep fascia. At the level of the fascia lata a finger extends the plane of dissection searching for perforating veins. This should be done gently but thoroughly.

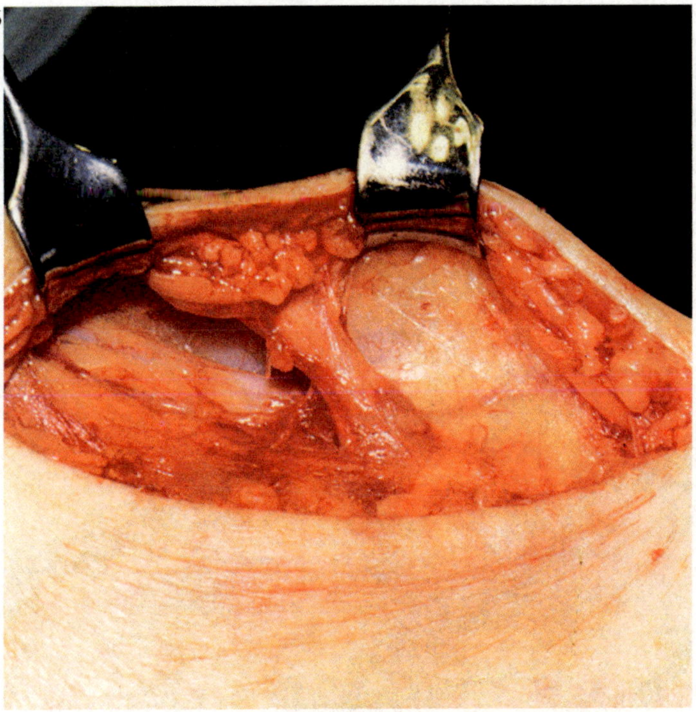

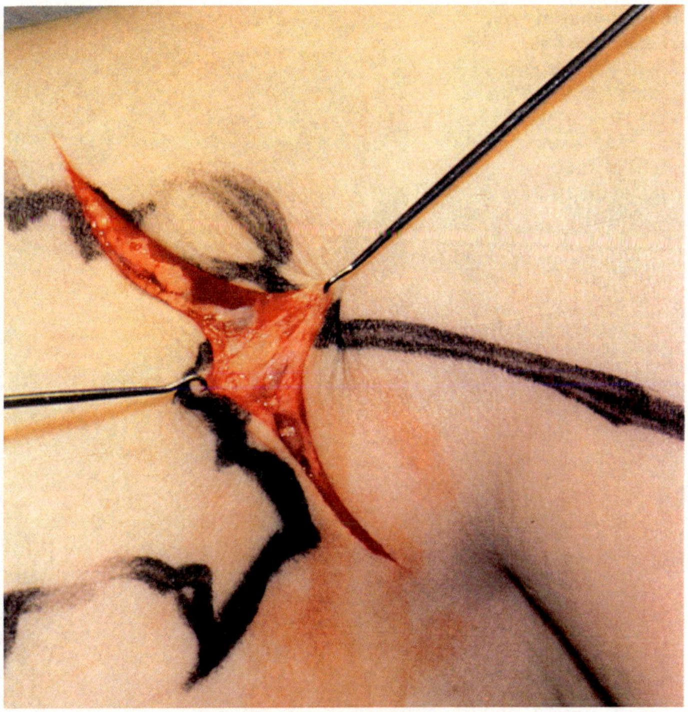

56 A perforator. Here a perforating vein is seen passing through an opening in the deep fascia. This is ligated flush with the deep fascia.

57 The knee incision. Just below the knee the LSV receives several tributaries, including the anterior and posterior arch veins. These are exposed through a skin crease incision. The wound edges are retracted with skin hooks.

58 Isolation of tributaries at the knee. The LSV is mobilised. Flexion of the knee helps the surgeon to free a substantial length of the vein, and to ligate the tributaries.

58

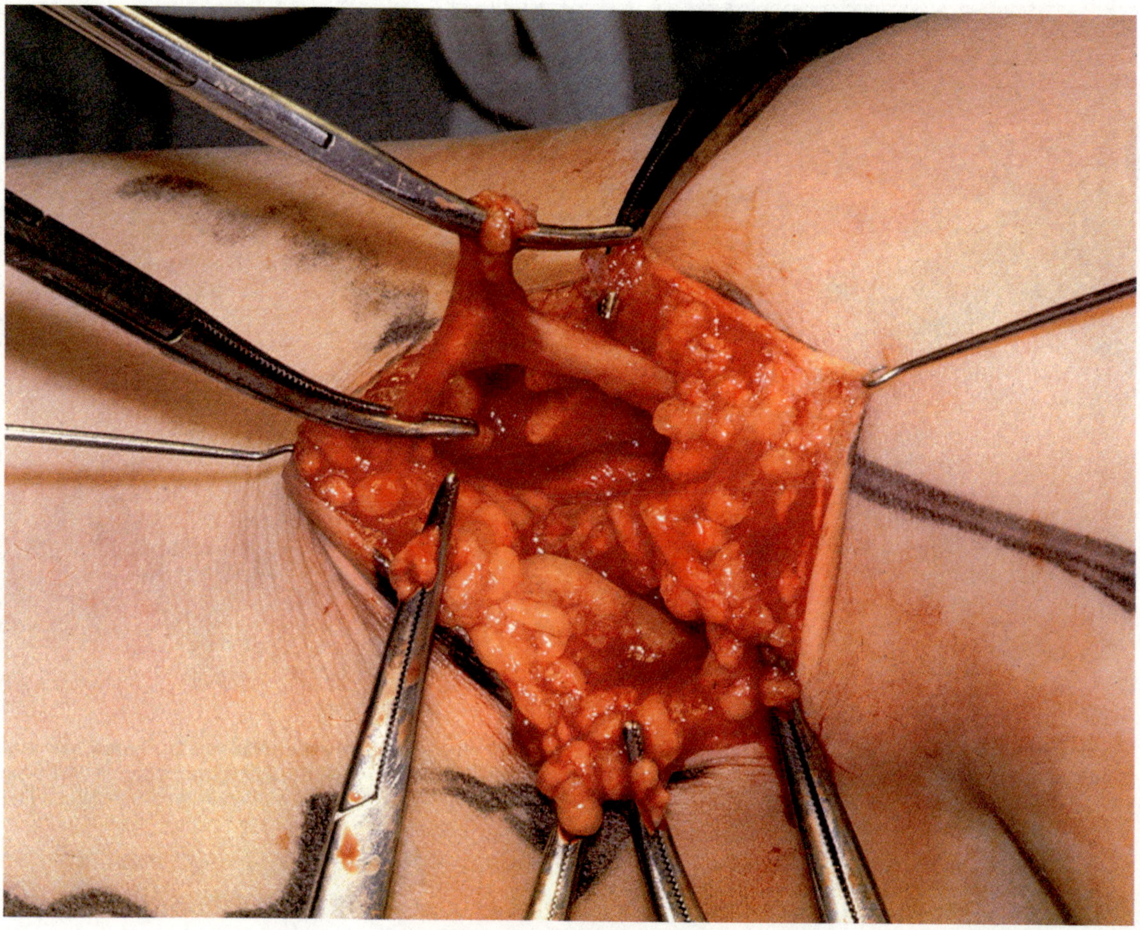

59 Wound closure. Careful skin apposition is important if a good cosmetic result is desired. Monofilament sutures are placed about a centimetre apart, without tension. They are removed on the twelfth postoperative day. Earlier removal of sutures in the calf can sometimes result in separation of the wound edges and unsightly scars.

59

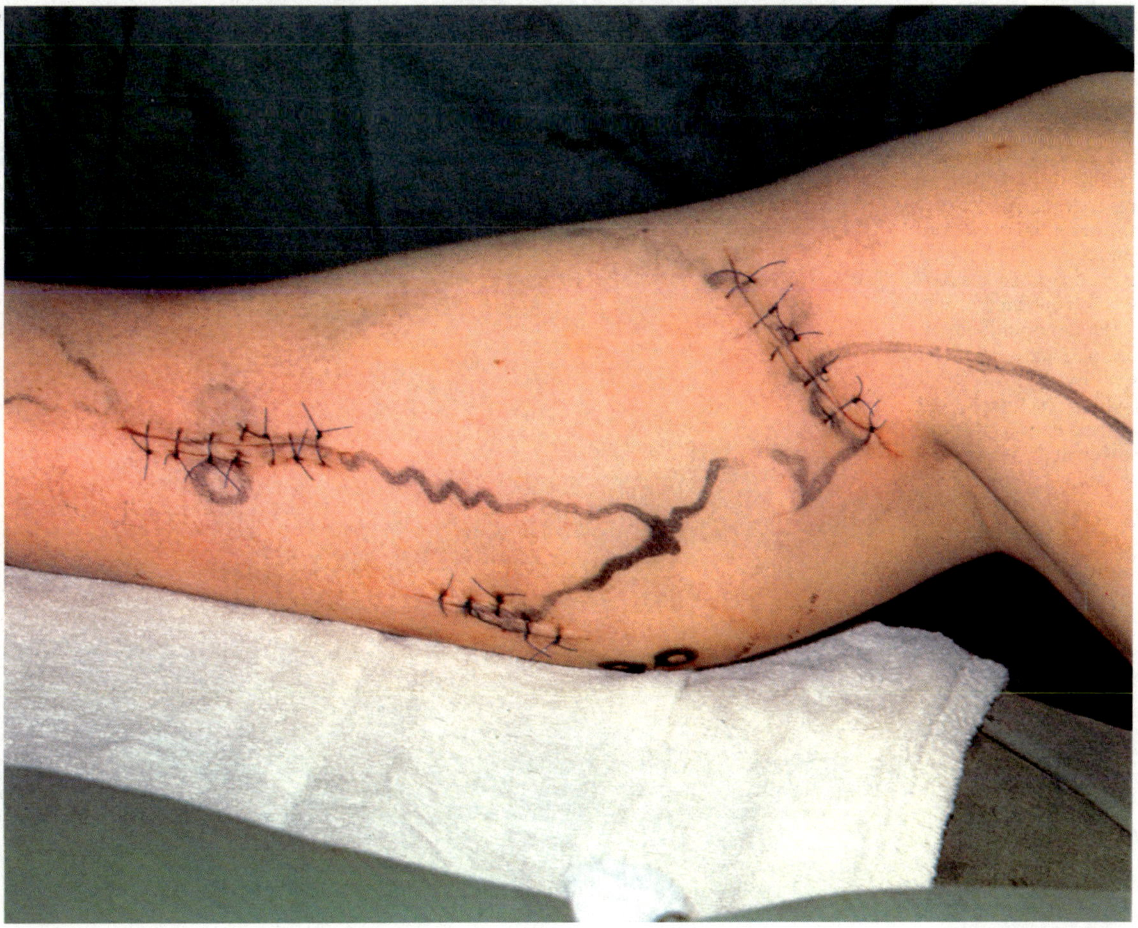

Avulsion

60
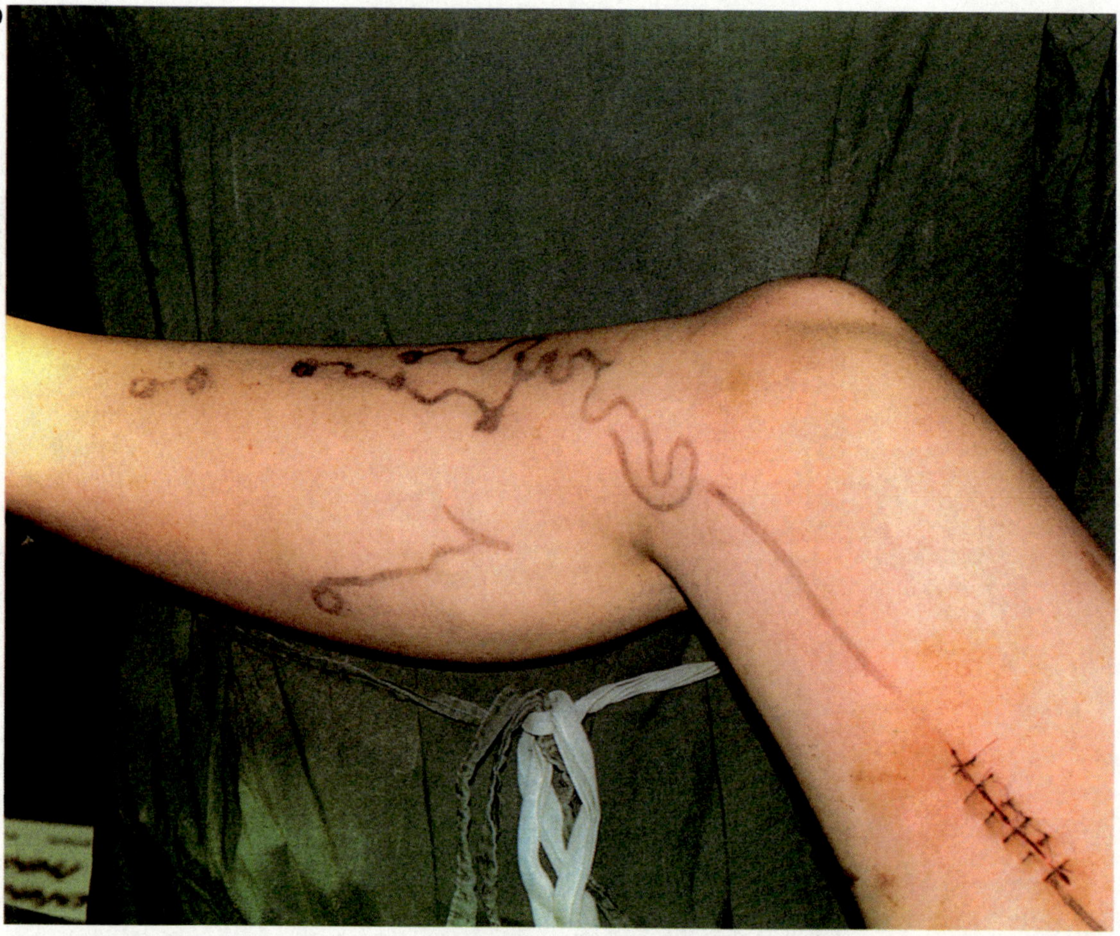

60 Avulsion method 1. This is an alternative technique for dealing with varicosities, especially below the level of the knee. It may be preferred when the patient is anxious to avoid scars, particularly if there is a keloid tendency. The leg is assessed and marked and saphenofemoral and/ or saphenopopliteal incompetence are dealt with by the dissection-ligation technique described earlier. The leg is elevated, held by the assistant.

61

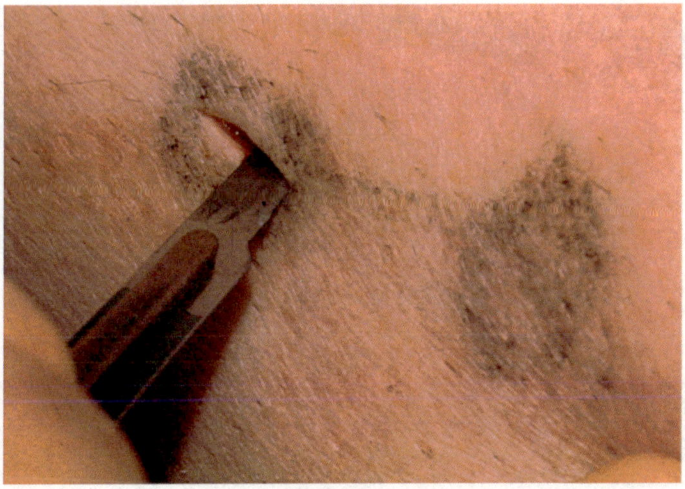

62

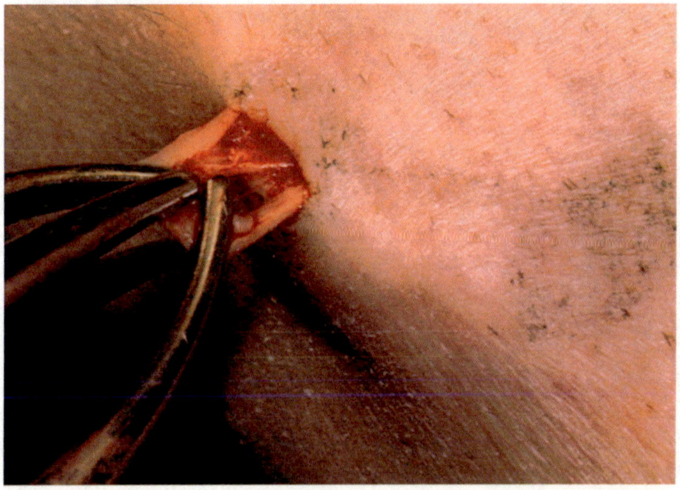

63

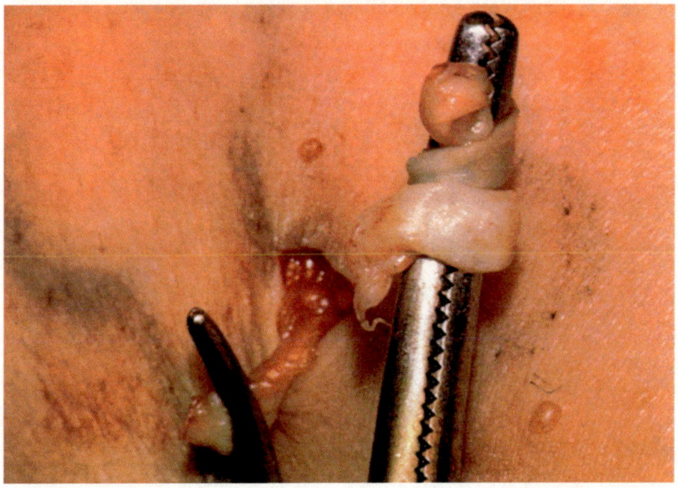

61 Avulsion method 2. A small stab incision is made over the varicosity.

62 Avulsion method 3. An artery forceps is inserted through the incision and the vein picked up. A second forceps is applied and the vein divided.

63 Avulsion method 4. By rotation of the forceps a segment of the vein is avulsed.

64

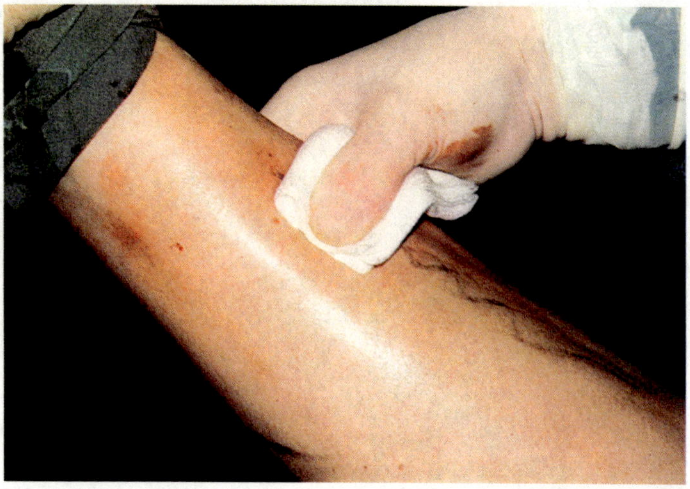

64 Avulsion method 5. Elevation of the leg and local compression ensure that there is minimal bleeding.

65

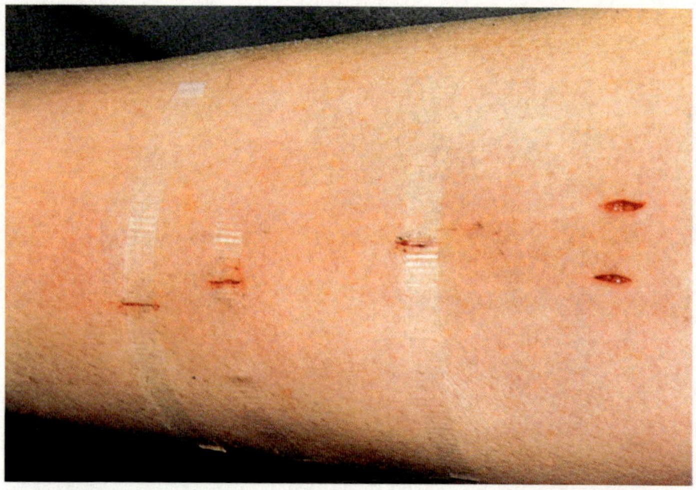

65 Avulsion method 6. The small incisions do not require suture. They can be closed with sterile adhesive strips. The leg is bandaged as described later.

Subfascial ligation

66

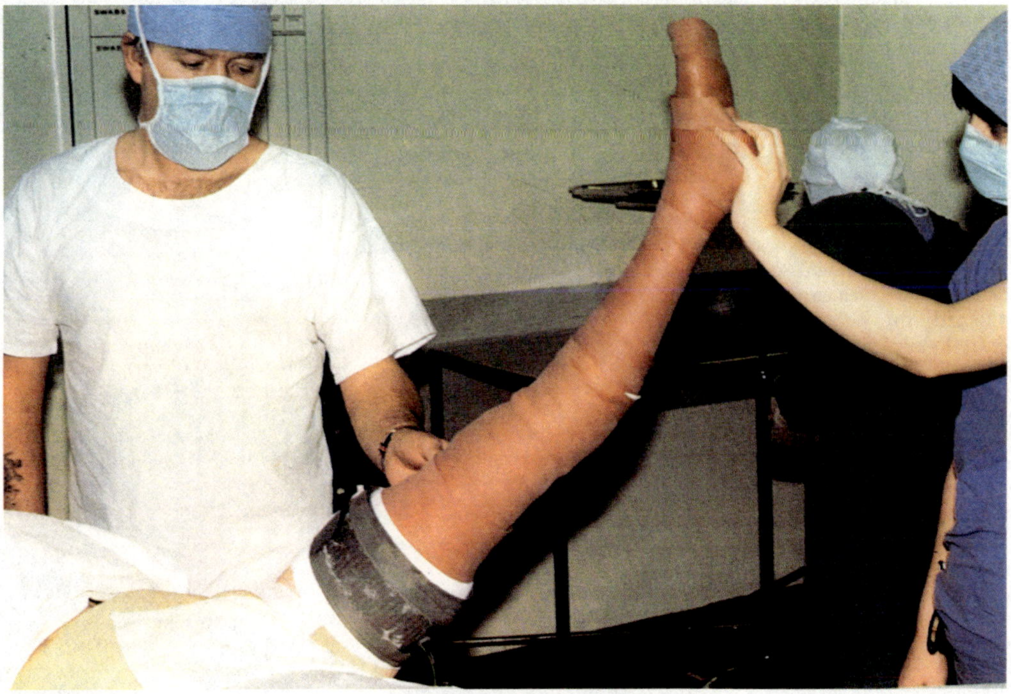

66 Subfascial ligation. Where it is decided to ligate perforating veins underneath the deep fascia a tourniquet is of value, especially where there is chronic inflammation and induration in the lower calf.

As a first stage, varicosities at a higher level are dealt with in routine fashion as described earlier. The wounds are closed and dressed. A tourniquet cuff is then applied around the thigh, and an Esmarch bandage is wound from the toes to empty the leg of blood.

67 The skin incision. The position of the incision depends on the site of the incompetent perforators and the pathological changes in the skin and subcutaneous tissues. A suitable incision is made at the medial border of soleus and carried down behind the posteromedial border of the tibia, but not beyond the medial malleolus. If tissues are inflamed or severely scarred a preferable incision is placed in the median line of the calf posteriorly and deviated medially off the Achilles tendon 3 to 4cm above the ankle joint. This incision allows access to both medial and latent perforators. The skin edges are retracted with skin hooks. No attempt is made to dissect subcutaneously. The incision is carried down and through the deep fascia.

67

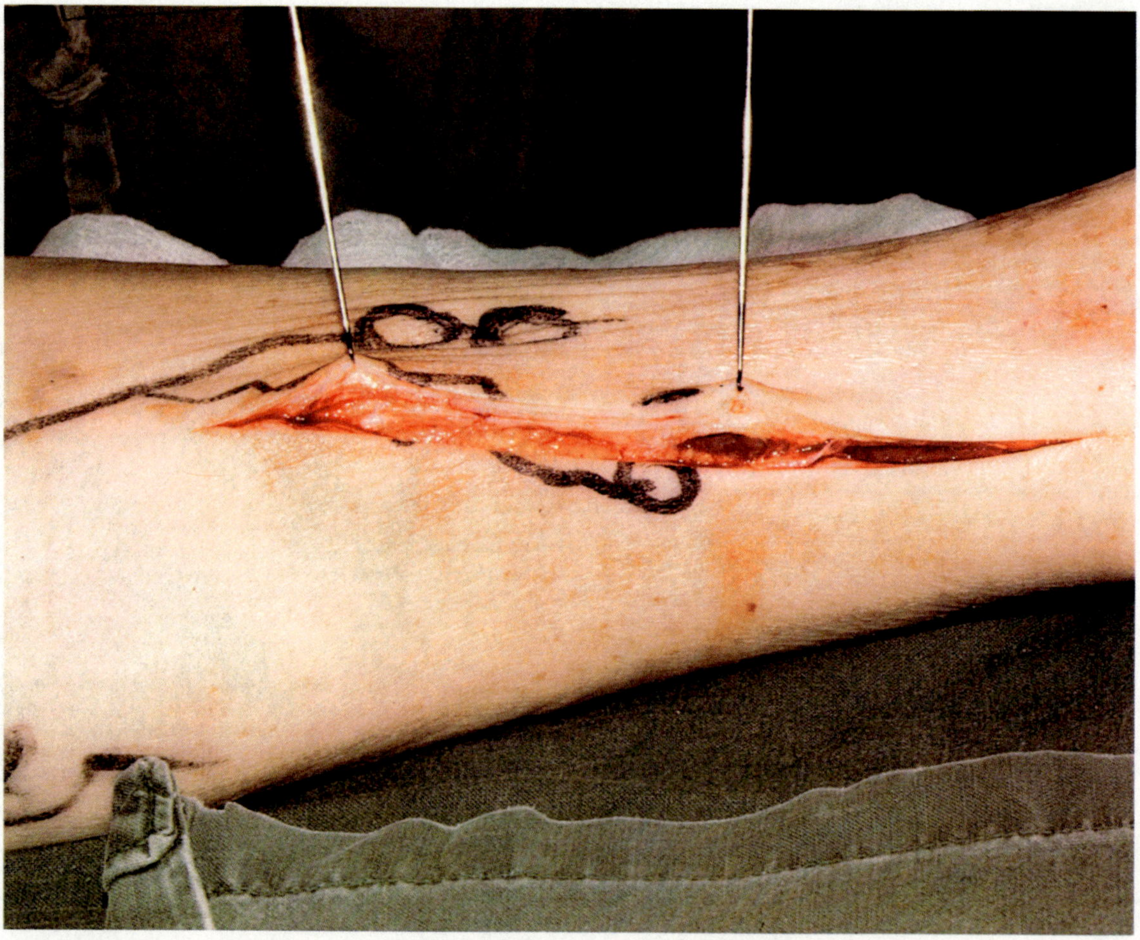

68 Subfascial dissection. No attempt is made to dissect out superficial veins which are simply ligated where they cross, the wound. The incision is carried down to and through the deep fascia which is raised off the muscle. Perforating veins can be seen penetrating the deep fascia.

68

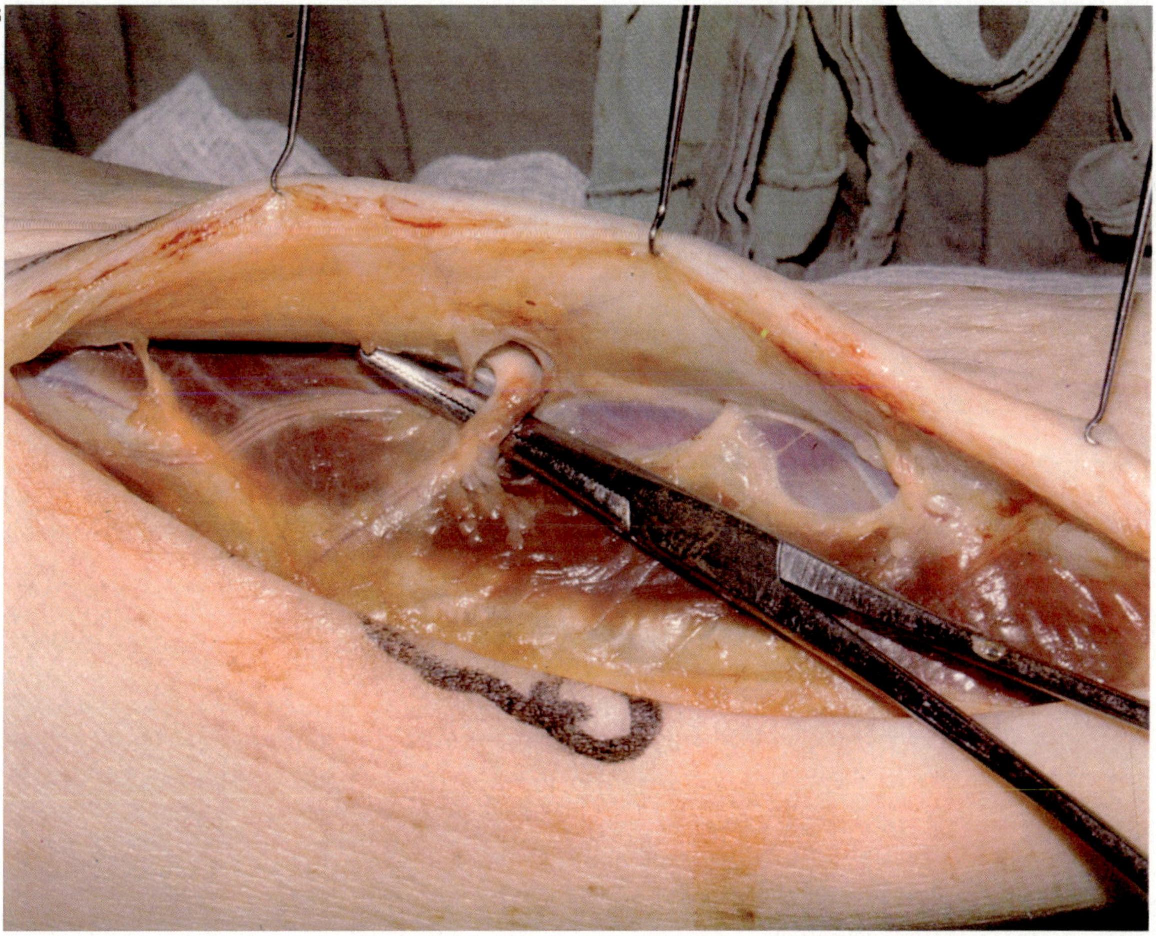

69

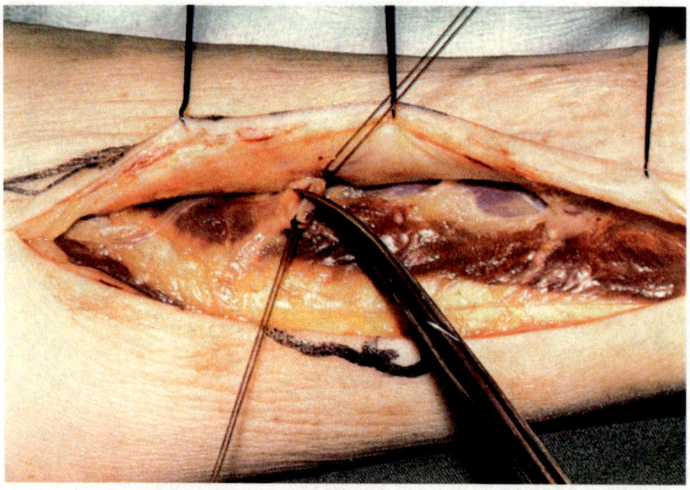

69 Ligation of perforators. Perforating veins are divided between catgut ligatures.

70

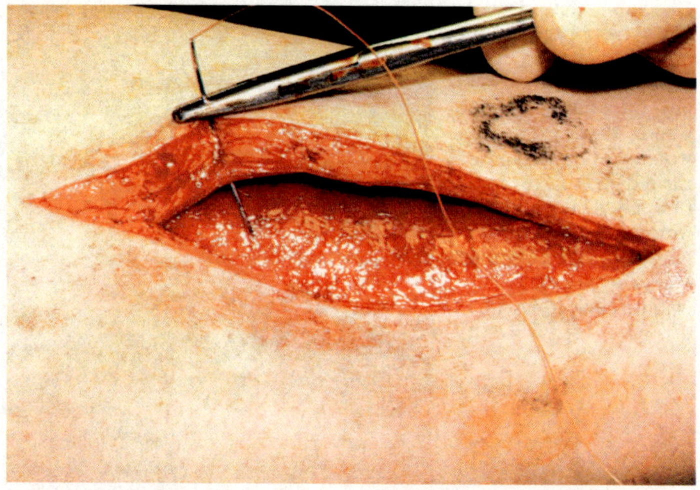

70 Closure of deep fascia. The deep fascia is restored with interrupted catgut sutures.

71 Wound closure. The wound is closed with interrupted polypropylene sutures. The tourniquet is not removed until dressings and compression bandaging has been completed.

71

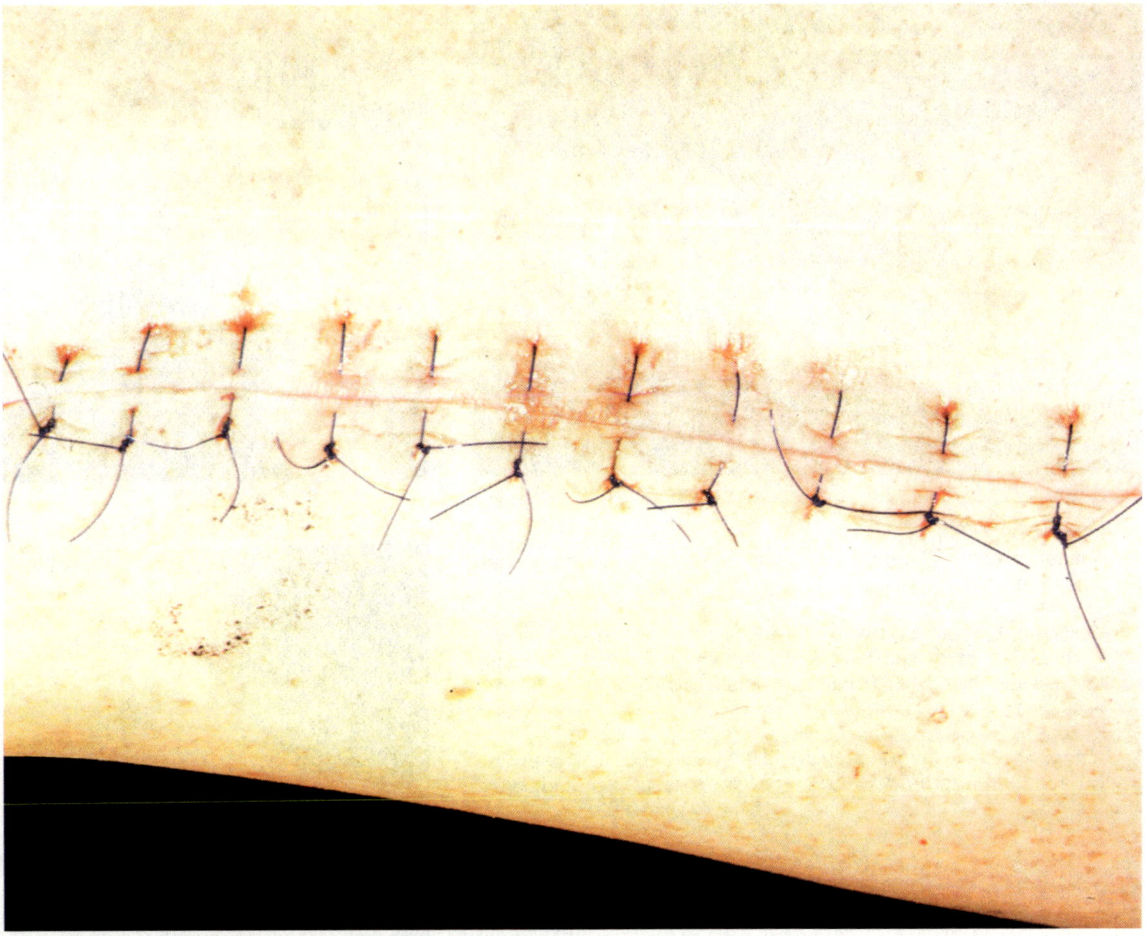

72 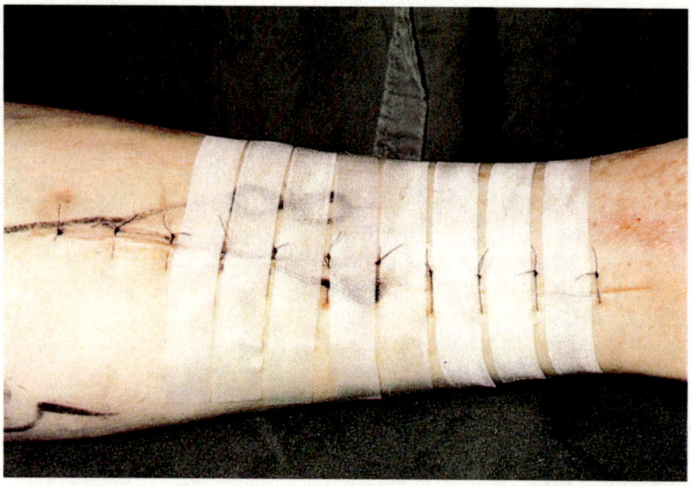

73 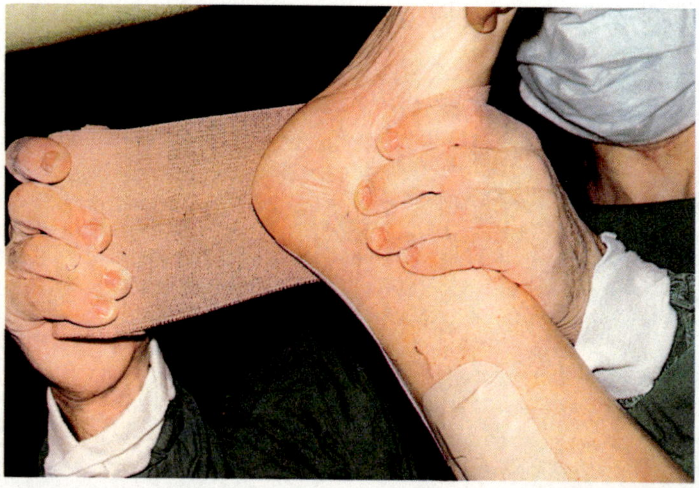

74 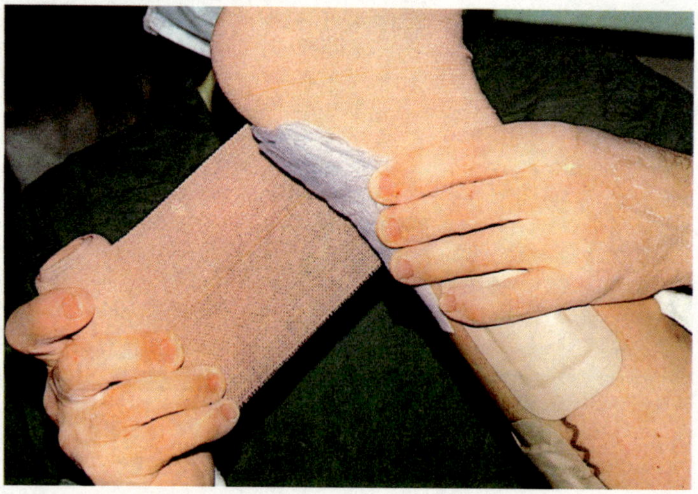

72 Wound closure. Wound tapes may be used to improve skin approximation.

73 Bandaging 1. Postoperative bandaging is important. A high quality elastic bandage is used – in this case Elastocrepe. The surgeon begins with a turn round the heel. The bandage is then carried down to the toes and back.

74 Bandaging 2. To avoid pressure damage to the skin over the Achilles tendon, a protective layer of gauze is placed under the bandage.

75

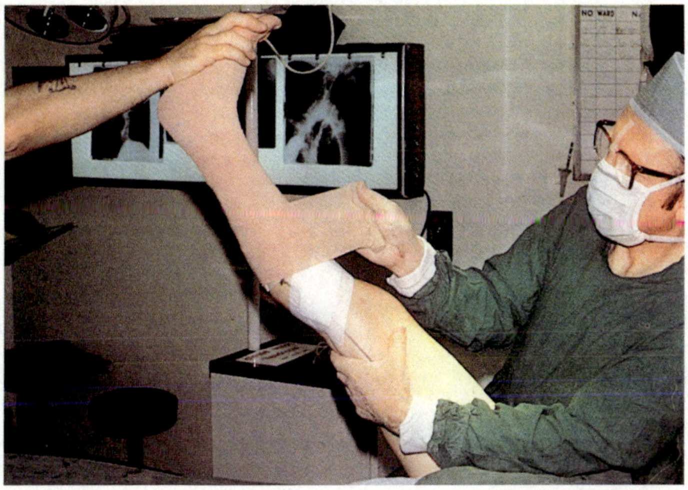

76

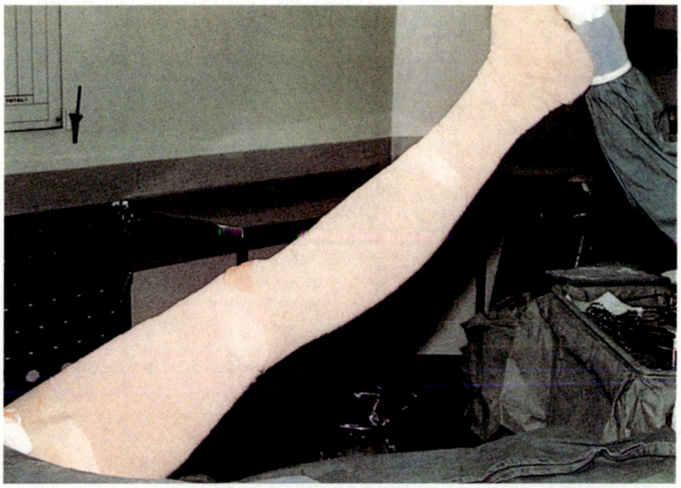

77

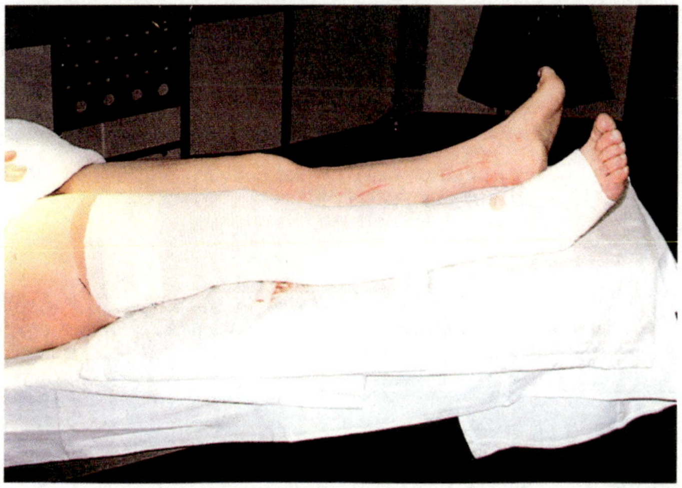

75 Bandaging 3. The bandaging continues firmly up the leg with sufficient overlap to give even compression. As with all elastic bandages, the compression should diminish as it ascends the leg.

76 Bandaging 4. A small gap is left at the front of the knee to allow flexion.

77 Bandaging 5. A graduated compression tubular bandage is then applied over the cotton crepe bandage. Note the strip of elastic surgical adhesive tape around the upper end to avoid rolling and the small hole at the front of the ankle to avoid pressure on extensor tendons. Alternatively a single layer of self-adhesive bandage may be used.

References

Fegan, W.G., 'Continuous compression technique of injecting varicose veins', *Lancet*, 1963, **ii**, 109-112.

Hobbs, J.T., 'Surgery and sclerotherapy in the treatment of varicose veins', *Arch. Surg.*, 1974, **109**,793-796.

Hobbs, J.T., 'Preoperative venography to ensure accurate saphenopopliteal vein ligation', *Brit. Med. J.*, 1981, **1**,1578-1579.

Linton, R.R., 'Surgery of veins of lower extremities', *Minn. Med.*, 1949, **32**,38-46.

Rivlin, S., 'The surgical cure of primary varicose veins', *Brit. J. Surg.*, 1975, **62**, 913-917.

Ruckley, C.V., Ludgate, C.M., MacLean, M. and Espley, A.J., 'Major outpatient surgery', *Lancet*, 1973, **ii**,1193-1196.

Ruckley, C.V., Cuthbertson, C., Fenwick, F., Prescott, R.J. and Garraway, W.M., 'Day care after operations for hernia or varicose veins: a controlled trial', *Brit. J. Surg.*, 1978, **65**,456-459.

Stephens, F.O. and Dudley, H.A.F., 'An organisation for outpatient surgery'. *Lancet*, 1973, **ii**,1042-1044.

Index

All numbers refer to page numbers.

Zeitfracht Medien GmbH
Ferdinand-Jühlke-Straße 7
99095 Erfurt, Deutschland
produktsicherheit@kolibri360.de